The Concept of *Botho* and HIV/AIDS in Botswana

Zapf Chancery Tertiary Level Publications

A Guide to Academic Writing by C. B. Peter (1994)

Africa in the 21st Century by Eric M. Aseka (1996)

Women in Development by Egara Kabaji (1997)

Introducing Social Science: A Guidebook by J. H. van Doorne (2000)

Elementary Statistics by J. H. van Doorne (2001)

Iteso Survival Rites on the Birth of Twins by Festus B. Omusolo (2001)

The Church in the New Millennium: Three Studies in the Acts of the Apostles by John Stott (2002)

Introduction to Philosophy in an African Perspective by Cletus N.Chukwu (2002)

Participatory Monitoring and Evaluation by Francis W. Mulwa and Simon N. Nguluu (2003)

Applied Ethics and HIV/AIDS in Africa by Cletus N. Chukwu (2003)

For God and Humanity: 100 Years of St. Paul's United Theological College Edited by Emily Onyango (2003)

Establishing and Managing School Libraries and Resource Centres by Margaret Makenzi and Raymond Ongus (2003)

Introduction to the Study of Religion by Nehemiah Nyaundi (2003)

A Guest in God's World: Memories of Madagascar by Patricia McGregor (2004)

Introduction to Critical Thinking by J. Kahiga Kiruki (2004)

Theological Education in Contemporary Africa edited by GrantLeMarquand and Joseph D. Galgalo (2004)

Looking Religion in the Eye edited by Kennedy Onkware (2004)

Computer Programming: Theory and Practice by Gerald Injendi (2005)

Demystifying Participatory Development by Francis W. Mulwa (2005)

Music Education in Kenya: A Historical Perspective by Hellen A. Odwar (2005)

Into the Sunshine: Integrating HIV/AIDS into Ethics Curriculum Edited by Charles Klagba and C. B. Peter (2005)

Integrating HIV/AIDS into Ethics Curriculum: Suggested Modules Edited by Charles Klagba (2005)

Dying Voice (An Anthropological Novel) by Andrew K. Tanui (2006)

Participatory Learning and Action (PLA): A Guide to Best Practice by Enoch Harun Opuka (2006)

Science and Human Values: Essays in Science, Religion, and Modern Ethical Issues edited by Nehemiah Nyaundi and Kennedy Onkware (2006)

Understanding Adolescent Behaviour by Daniel Kasomo (2006)

Students' Handbook for Guidance and Counselling by Daniel Kasomo (2007)

BusinessOrganization an Management: Questions and Answers by Musa O. Nyakora (2007)

Auditing Priniples: A Stuents' Handbook by Musa O. Nyakora (2007)

The Concept of Botho and HIV/AIDS in Botswana edite by Joseph B. R. Gaie and Sana K. MMolai (2007)

The Concept of *Botho* and HIV/AIDS in Botswana

Edited by
Joseph B. R. Gaie, PhD
Sana K. MMolai, PhD

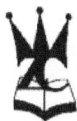

Zapf Chancery
Eldoret, Kenya

First Published 2007
© Joseph B. R. Gaie and Sana K. MMolai
All rights reserved.

Cover prodution team
Joseph B. R. Gaie, C. B. Peter, and Michael Chege

Copyeditor
R. Venkatasamy, PhD

Associate Designer
Mihael Nchimbi

Publishing Consultant
C. B. Peter

Printed by
Kijabe Printing Press,
P. O. Box 40,
Kijabe.

Published by

Zapf Chancery Research Consultants and Publishers,
P. O. Box 4988,
Eldoret, Kenya.
Email: zapfchancerykenya@yahoo.co.uk
Mobile: 0721-222 311 or 0733-915 814

ISBN 9966-7185-5-9

*This book is printed on fully recyclable,
environment-friendly paper.*

To Billy Mosedame, Cynthia Leshomo, and all the other great warriors in the struggle against HIV and AIDS, all those who are fighting the virus now, those who have told the world about it and a host of other unsung heroines and heroes of our nation and other nations of the world.

And

To the great sages of our beloved Botswana who have bequeathed us with the great Setswana wisdom and language.

Joseph B. R. Gaie
Sana K. MMolai

Great warriors who fought
The gallant fight against the big
Enemy HIV, you are our pride
You are our salvation
You are our teachers
You are the toast of
Your nations
the divinity
Of our souls.

Great warriors fighting the fight now
We are proud of you, we love you
We respect you, we will always admire you
Courage! Hold your heads high for your salvation is near
Be of good cheer for each of us is just like you
We will never die for death is but an illusion.

We are made of divine stuff
We are divinity itself
Our love will always shine through
And thus teach us that we will never die
For death has been forever condemned
To the world of illusions.

In the world of the living there is neither
Sickness nor hunger
Pain and suffering are illusory
They are replaced by the apparently
Illusory definite real eternity
Take heart my love, take heart
We are in this together
Our love will see us through

-Joseph Balatedi Radinkudikae Gaie

Acknowledgements

We are happy to acknowledge the support of Lebani Duncan Mokhuni, Teddy Onkabetse Rahube for their support in collecting data for Chapter four of this book. We would also like to thank other participants, informants and facilitators for the researches that led to all the chapters of this book. We are forever grateful to our nation for the great opportunity accorded us in all the different aspects of our lives.

We thank all our sources for availing the information that we have used to us and the rest of the world.

We have made every attempt to acknowledge and trace all copyright material. Any omission to acknowledge our sources is inadvertent, and we shall be pleased to correct it, should it be pointed out to us.

Finally, we are grateful to our publishers, Zapf Chancery Research Consultants and Publishers, PO Box 4988, Eldoret, Kenya, the entire publishing team, and espeially the Rev. C. B. Peter, Founder and Senior Publishing Consultant, Zapf Chancery, for publishing this book.

Table of Contents

Introduction

Joseph B. R. Gaie

The context of HIV&AIDS is that there has been a debate, or rather an assumption or assumptions as to where the disease belongs. Is it just a medical problem that needs medical solutions, or is there much more to it than that? Those of us who reflect on these matters soon realise that no disease is just a medical problem. As long as it affects human beings, there will always be social, cultural, political, economic, ethical, anthropological, psychological, and sociological aspects that are crucial in dealing with the disease. Thus, this book brings a dimension that many might not think as being important in understanding the importance of different aspects of society in so far as it relates to HIV and AIDS.

This book is about the concept of *Botho* (Humanhood) amongst the *Batswana* (the people of Botswana) during the HIV&AIDS pandemic. The book will endeavour to analyse and establish the implications of HIV&AIDS for *Botho* as a concept on the one hand, and the implications of *Botho* for HIV&AIDS on the other hand.

This book has been divided into seven chapters. The first chapter will define and analyse the Setswana concept of *Botho* from a theological perspective. The chapter is intended to help the reader to understand how the concept of *Botho* can be understood from the Christian perspective. It will start by relating the concept of *Botho* with the divinity of God within humankind, as depicted in the Bible.

Chapter one will also compare and contrast the theology of "holiness being communal wholeness," as depicted in the spirituality of *Botho*, with the Christian concept of love and human divinity. In this connection, the chapter will argue that both concepts are similar and are crucial in caring for those infected and affected by HIV&AIDS. The chapter will further contextualize the theological implications of HIV&AIDS in an African setting for both the infected and the affected. It will be argued that the spirituality of *Botho* and the Christian concept of love are the key concepts in understanding and combating gender and socio-economic inequalities related to HIV&AIDS.

The second chapter will explore the multifaceted Setswana concept of *Botho*. It will begin by critically analyzing the metaphysical and epistemological aspects of *Botho*, and how this concept is related to love, compassion, and morality. The chapter will also explore the morality aspect of *Botho*, by relating it to current obstacles of HIV&AIDS in Botswana. The chapter will further illustrate how the concept of *Botho* is universal and present in other African cultures.

The third chapter will look at various ways in which the maid is disadvantaged economically, as compared to other workers. The chapter will use the *Botho* framework to show how failure to practice *Botho* directly or indirectly contributes to the HIV&AIDS pandemic. The chapter will illustrate the situation of a maid by arguing that whilst the maid is expected to show the very best attributes of humanity, she is not afforded the same by her employers.

It will be argued that in general, whilst on the one hand the maid does not disclose their HIV&AIDS status to the employer for fear of losing the job, on the other hand the family also does not disclose their HIV status. The chapter will demonstrate how the maid is forced by economic reasons to risk her life where HIV&AIDS is concerned. This chapter will further argue that people's rights should cease to be rights if they impinge on other people's rights.

The fourth chapter will explore and analyze cultural beliefs, practices and understandings that influence people's perceptions of various notions. It will demonstrate how the cultural and religious beliefs of Batswana directly influence their understanding about HIV&AIDS. For instance, it will be illustrated how Batswana seem to associate HIV&AIDS with *Boswagadi* (widowhood), so that they can deal with HIV&AIDS easily because the symptoms of both are similar. Against this background, the chapter will argue that it will be difficult for the people to let go of their cultural and religious beliefs when faced with new situations.

The chapter will maintain that there is a need to understand and appreciate that some of the Batswana's religious and cultural beliefs and practices enrich their understanding of HIV&AIDS. The central argument of this chapter will be that *Botho* demands us to acknowledge and appreciate people's religious and cultural beliefs and practices. This acknowledgement, as will be demonstrated, will be an empowerment in the fight against HIV&AIDS.

This chapter will further examine some cultural and religious practices, which block the fight against HIV&AIDS. The chapter will endeavor to illustrate how it would be impossible to discard such cultural practices without affecting other important concepts of the people, such as *Botho*.

The aim of the fifth chapter will be to explore and establish the implications of the methods to combat HIV&AIDS for *Botho*. The chapter will start by arguing that abstinence before marriage promotes *Botho,* even though condomisation seems to be given priority over abstinence. It will be maintained that despite the fact that the traditional attitude is for spouses (especially husbands) to have extra-marital affairs, faithfulness to one's partner is consistent with *Botho*.

It will be argued that the use of condoms is likely to encourage people to have multiple partners. This method, it will be illustrated, may also lead children to engage in sexual intercourse at a very young age. It will also be argued that the use of condoms can be an empowerment for commercial sex workers. The chapter will further argue that whilst condomisation is given priority over other methods used to combat HIV&AIDS, it is inconsistent with *Botho*.

The sixth chapter will analyze the role of education in transmitting acceptable behavior in classical, traditional, and modern societies. The chapter will specifically explore the role of religious education in promoting *Botho*. Specifically, the chapter will illustrate the role played by religious education (within any education system) in promoting acceptable behaviors of the learners. It will start by showing how African traditional education used religion to transmit values associated with responsible sexual behavior. This, it will be demonstrated, helped in the reduction of illicit sexual relationships amongst boys and girls.

The chapter will also show how the Christian missionaries who introduced education in Africa ensured that religious education was part of the curriculum due to its contribution in promoting moral development. The chapter will further show how religious education can promote acceptable behaviors among Botswana secondary school students. The chapter will maintain that since religious education lays emphasis on acceptable behavior, it is capable of promoting *Botho*, and this can help in the control of the spread of HIV&AIDS.

The seventh and final chapter focuses on whether or not it is acceptable for prospective students to be tested for HIV&AIDS prior to scholarship grants. The chapter will begin by arguing the immorality of compulsory HIV&AIDS testing, and differentiates this morality from a situation in which the scholarship is made dependent on a negative HIV&AIDS test with a student's full consent.

The chapter will maintain that the latter situation is morally acceptable. Using utilitarian and Kantian arguments, this position will be argued and consolidated by highlighting the role of justifiable violation of human rights. Central to the argument of the chapter will be that HIV&AIDS testing is consistent with the Setswana concept of *Botho*.

CHAPTER ONE

Botho and HIV&AIDS: A Theological Reflection

Dumi Oafeta Mmualefhe

God as being-itself is the ground of every relation; in his life, all relations are present beyond the distinction between potentiality and actuality. However, they are not the relations of God with something else. They are the inner relations of the divine life

(Tillich, 1967: 271)

Botho: A Definition

*B*otho is an answer to the question: "What is authentic humanity?" *Botho*, at face value, is a *Sotho-Tswana* equivalent of the English word "person", so *Botho* can in the same way be translated to mean personhood. The Sotho-Tswana language groups, found mainly in Botswana, South Africa, and Lesotho, are part of a larger group spreading from Eastern Nigeria through the Cameroon, Congo, Kenya, Angola, and the rest of Southern Africa, called *Bantu (*King, 1970:32). *Botho*, among the Nguni language groups in Southern Africa, and among most other groups throughout Africa, is known as *Ubuntu. Ubuntu* is in fact a generic word used by the Bantu people of Africa. *Ubuntu* and *Botho* can therefore be used interchangeably.

It is difficult to say with certainty what the root *–ntu* means. The root*–ntu* with the prefix: *mu-* forms the singular *muntu*; the plural on the other hand would use the prefix *ba-* to form *Bantu*, which is loosely translated as people. *Ubuntu* carries the same root, *–ntu* prefixed with *ubu-*denoting a particular way of doing things which reflects true humanness or personhood.

According to Booth (1977: 35), the Baluba tribe of the Congo uses the same root with a prefix *ki-* for a thing. One can therefore argue that being Bantu themselves, the usage of the prefix *ubu-* would point to a particular way of doing things, that makes a thing to reflect true humanness.

Ray (2000: 10-120) records a Baganda mythology of the origins of life and death. The Baganda are a Bantu group found in the present day Uganda. In their mythology, Kintu was the first man who wandered alone in the vast plains of the country of Baganda. He met a woman who, together with her brother, came from the sky. The woman, Nnambi, took an immediate liking for Kintu. He left with her to meet *Ggulu*, Nnambi's father, in the sky, where Kintu asked her father for Nnambi's hand in marriage. They married and had many children. Death came through the evil Walumbe (death), Nnambi's brother. Kintu's children however multiplied. As the story goes, Kintu's last words were, "The descendent of Kintu will never die out!" (Ray, 2000:10-12).

The point of this myth, like its biblical counterpart, is the relationship humanity has with God, which is similar to what is believed in *Setswana*. Like in Setswana, God is the creator of human beings. In addition to the question of creation, the story sheds some light on the issue of good and evil. Whenever calamities like HIV&AIDS befall us, we cannot help but ask questions like, "if God is indeed almighty, then how do we account for evil and the pain that we endure?" Whenever we feel death knocking on our doors, we start wondering as to how to account for this "evil."

According to this Baganda mythology, human anxieties and disobedience have led to the co-existence of good and evil.

The Baganda's account of creation is important in that it binds God, humanity, and the whole creation into a relational communion. This communion is necessary for the wellness and wholeness of creation, and this includes especially human beings. The Bantu commonly believe that the breach of this all-important relationship brings about disease and death. Batswana have always viewed sickness as being a result of estrangement. In the Baganda creation myth, Walumbe is an estranged son who brings death upon Kintu's children. Whereas the story recognizes the reality of death, it is not clouded with sheer pessimism. Bantu have always been sustained by hope, even against hope. Even in the midst of death the myth ends with an assurance of life, that the "descendents of Kintu will never die". Setswana will in the same way say "*go swa motho go sale motho,*" that is, whenever a person dies, there is always someone remaining. Death, in an African setting, is defeated by the very relational nature of the so called profane and divine. In fact, the absence or the downplaying of dichotomies brings about a sense of continuation, which is only experienced in communal relationships. This is a different worldview from the mainstream Western tradition.

Botho emphasizes relationships; it is about concern for others. *Motho* is a 'relating thing.' The very definition of what *Motho* is cannot be divorced from the existence and the well-being of others. One's definition of well-being therefore depends on the being and well-being of others in the spirit of "I relate, therefore, I am". Mbiti avers syllogistically that *Motho* is one who is "conscious of himself in terms of "I am because we are, and since we are, therefore I am" (Mbiti, 1970:282). One's ability or inability to relate to others therefore is fundamental to his or her definition as a *Motho*. Needless to say, the inability to relate will relegate a human being to something less than a *Motho*.

"The Descendents of Kintu will never die out!"

Life, by nature (whatever that means) is paradoxically terminal. No wonder someone said, "Life is a terminal disease transmitted through sexual intercourse." Death is therefore the terminal point of life, which does not at the same time spell the end of the same life. It is at times called the most common denominator that is no respecter of status. John Hick writes:

> Death comes impartially to everyone; there are no privileged or underprivileged in this matter; we are all in the end in the same boat, together not only with our contemporaries but also with our ancestors and all our descendants.
>
> (Hick, 1976:87)

Death here, I would propose, is the clinical demise of being, and indeed a culmination of human temporality. In death, we see the end of our temporal being. This temporal being is the visible part of a *Motho,* that is, the body. This leads to my second proposal, and that is, in spite of its imposing finality, death for an African, as is the case with many other peoples of the world, is not the end of being. It is because of this conviction that, as Africans, we join each other and in unison declare; "The descendents of Kintu will never die out" song!

My intention and mission is, however, not to talk about death, but instead to talk about life. To talk about HIV&AIDS is not to talk about death, but about life, as those infected are those who still live amongst us. To talk about HIV&AIDS in the context of *Botho* is to engage in a serious spiritual introspection. It is about looking deeply into the meaning of "I am because we are", which transcends the physical world, but most importantly, includes the "cloud of witnesses" that always encompass us (Hebrews 12:1). Talking about HIV&AIDS is about engaging ourselves in a reality check; it is to place ourselves into "the bigger picture" in order to determine where we stand, who we are, for what purpose we live, and most importantly, what we are! To address this issue is to focus on **us,** and not **them**, for in *Botho* there is no **them**. We can talk about **them** only in so far as our 'identifiability' and identity as *Batho* depends on the **BE-ness** of those we erroneously regard as "them, those, and others!"

I elected to start by mentioning death because whenever HIV&AIDS is mentioned, our brains and emotions switch into the "death gear." Some even look at the infected as *Bo moipolai ba ba sa lelelweng,* that is, those who called death upon themselves. Most importantly, those infected are discriminated against, they suffer stigma as they are viewed as "those who called death upon themselves." I want to propose that this is not only an issue of theological interest, but also that our **BE-ness,** and our ultimate relationship with the divine hinges upon it. Life, or rather conception, is possible because of *Botho*-pre-natal activity. I am here not talking about the sexual encounter, but that which follow this encounter. The selflessness that *Botho* is about is perfectly demonstrated in the very process of conception. Hick, (1976: 36) observes that millions of spermatozoa are deposited into the vagina, yet only one would swim through. The interesting thing is that the success of one that proceeds to fertilize the ovum depends on the self-sacrifice of others along the "life-path." It is in this regard that he concludes:

> Nevertheless, this vast number is apparently needed. A single sperm, unsupported by its million companions, would not be able to make its way across the mucus area at the entry of the uterus, up the fallopian tube, and through the membrane protecting the egg, for each sperm produces only a minute quantity of the enzyme which digests the material to be penetrated, and it is only the combined action of the many that a way is made through the target. Thus, hundreds of millions of sperm perish in enabling one of their number to continue in the life of a new organism
>
> (Hick, 1976:36).

In the same way, life is sustained by working together, through the self-sacrifice of some for others, and others for some. It is this comradeship, this covenantal connectedness, and this commensality of *communitas,* which pours aspersion on the finality of death in the African context. There is, therefore, no room for "every man for himself and God for us all," as God cannot but be for those who relate. Our relationality with each other is therefore indivisible from our relationship with the divine; this is the spiritual meaning of *Botho*.

The Task of Theology of *Botho*

For theology to be meaningful at all, it must reflect and embrace what David Ford calls "ecology of responsibility" (Ford, 1999:18). It must address all spheres of life. This is not a kind of theology that is toyed with by those in academia; it ought to reflect on the religious community, and most importantly, on the society or the community within which the religious and academic communities reside. Furthermore, this theology, while not compromising its critical analytical and critical scholarly character, must be articulated "in the clearest and most coherent language available" (Macquarrie, 1977: 2). And I dare add, it must be coherent to the communities within which it is articulated. Such theology must be a lived theology, one that shares the breath of people who live it.

This would bring another challenge: the problem of theological language. The challenge, I would propose, is to enrich it by embracing the language of the host community or communities. We therefore should not shy away from introducing, for instance, Setswana words, especially those that may not have English equivalents, into theological discourse. If need be, new words ought to be created to expand theological vocabulary. This would be nothing new, as life has always dictated that as life unfolds, language should expand. True theology thrives on adaptation.

Botho, as alluded to, is a spiritual concept, and therefore of theological interest. *Botho* is that **Godness** in the Bantu that touches on the whole of their being and existence. *Botho* is that glory of divinity that radiates from Bantu/*Batho*. This glory manifests itself in their connectedness. Prof. Gabriel Setiloane uses the Setswana metaphor of *Seriti* to point to the spirituality and divinity of *Botho*. I hasten to point out that this *Seriti* is different from one usually talked about when referring to some as having *seriti;* "so and so *o na le seriti*" as this translates to "so and so has charisma." This *seriti* does not refer to charisma. He defines this *seriti*, which has the same root as *mo-riti that* is shade and shadow as:

> a physical phenomenon, which expresses itself externally to the human body in a dynamic manner. It is like an aura around the human person, an invisible shadow, or cloud, or mist forming something like a magnetic or radar field.
>
> (Setiloane, 1986:13).

Seriti is that which has some effect on those around one, on the community, at the same time that which forms a community, which makes *Batho* see in one *motho* or *phologolo* (person or animal).

Motho ought to have *seriti* which is to a person what a magnetic field is to a magnet. It is this "magnetic field" that draws a line in defining one metal object from others. Without it, the matter is but a metal, and it is only with this "field" that this metal becomes a force that can pull or repel other metals. This "field" energizes and vitalizes the otherwise dead metal, setting it apart from other inactive metals and objects. A magnet, being filled with vitality, brings about activity not only on itself, but moves other metal objects around it into activity.

Seriti is the energy that exudes from one without which one is dead, or rather, is not *motho*. *Seriti* is a connecting force that brings the community together, that attracts what is good, and repels what is bad. One with *seriti* is loving and selfless. *Seriti* is the vital force that makes one to see oneself in terms of and through others. *Seriti* makes the individual "conscious of himself in terms of 'I am because we are, and since we are, therefore I am'" (Mbiti, 1970:282).

Setiloane opines that this energy that exudes from one is the *kabod*, usually presented in religious art as a luminous ring that hangs over the heads of the saintly.

The radiance of 'Seriti', and I presume similarly of 'kabod' in man and in Divinity exudes itself through the whole. For God it literally means everything, in and through everything in the whole creation (Psalm 139:18). That is why it is transferable. [...] It is this kind of experience an African understands Jesus was going through in Luke 8: 45-46: '[...] someone has touched me; for I perceive that power has gone forth from me.'

(Setiloane, 1986:14).

Theology concerns itself with relationships. It analytically deals with relationships and articulations of the same. *Botho*, as a theological concept, views the whole life as relational. This resonates with Christianity which, when understood the Jesus' way, is based on love. When asked about which is the greatest commandment, Jesus points to the command to love God as the greatest, followed by one about loving one's neighbour. With these relational commandments, the rest is but commentary (Matt. 22:34-40). Here, Jesus challenges people to love until it bleeds, indeed to follow the example of the self-sacrificing millions of sperms!

The command to love one's neighbour is of paramount importance so much that the writer of the first epistle of John states that God is Love, and that to know God is to love, to not love, on the other hand, is to not know God. The writer further states that loving God, whom we cannot see, hinges on our loving those we see (1John 4:7-8, 20). "Love" here can be replaced with "relate" in the sense of *Botho*, hence *Motho ke motho ka batho*!(a person is a person through and with others) To know God is to relate. Those who do not relate therefore do not know God since God is relational. God is a covenantal God, and one cannot covenant alone. "Relate," like "love," is an active verb, both denote activity; they are action-oriented. Loving and relating are not about simply knowing each other: they go beyond the cognitive and emotive, they are spiritual, they are existential, and are about divine activity. It must be noted that relating here does not only refer to human beings, but to the whole creation, which translates into relating with the divine as per Paul Tillich's quotation at the beginning of this chapter.

Theological Implications of *Botho* for HIV&AIDS

In his "Letter from Birmingham City Jail," Martin Luther King Jr. writes:

> We are caught in an inescapable network of mutuality, tied in a single garment of destiny. Whatever affects one directly affects all indirectly.
>
> (Washington, 1986:290).

When greetings are exchanged, one often hears "*ga re a tsoga*" (we are not well). This does not mean the whole family is unwell, it could mean one of the family, relatives, or a member of the *kgotla* (ward/cell) is not well. When one is affected, we are all affected. Even more interestingly, when a traditional doctor is called, the divination is never individualized.

Illness has always been understood in a communal sense. Often, sickness would be attributed to *kgaba* (some kind of curse which befalls one who neglects his/her responsibility to care for, say a child, a relative or what belongs to the family). It could also be because of witchcraft, a result of strained relationships, or natural causes attributed to God. Both examples given above are respecters of neither political boundaries nor of distance, as they are spiritual reactions. Interestingly, HIV&AIDS was, and still is understood by some to be *boswagadi* (a condition one gets when they have had sexual intercourse with a widow or widower before the time of mourning has lapsed). In all these, it is the community that is ill, not just the individual. As a result, to bring healing, which could be in terms of bringing in a traditional doctor, or through sacrifices, is always communal. We are connected by the *Botho* magnetic force that draws us to one another.

An HIV positive member of a family is an HIV positive family; an HIV positive family is an HIV positive *kgotla*, village or town, and indeed the nation. This therefore rules out "her, him, and them!" We are in this together, we are all sick. To dispute this would be to do the same to our *Botho*, and therefore our spirituality. *Botho* is spiritual because for the Bantu, holiness is wholeness, since "the sacred is manifested not so much by separation as by unity. In Africa, it is undoubtedly true that the whole is the holy. Thus, man finds his fulfilment not as a separate individual, but as a participant in a family and a community" (Booth, 1977:7). It is together with the HIV positive that we are whole and therefore holy. In other words, salvation for the Bantu takes place in the context of community; it can only be understood in terms of the "preservation of a sense of communal wholeness" (Booth, 1977:9), while that which negates salvation, which is sin, "indicates a violation of relationships, resulting from alienation from God, nature, one another, and the self"(Suchocki, 1967:14).

St. Paul uses the body metaphor for the Church. He reflects the connectedness and relatedness of members of a body. He asks rhetorically: "If we all were a single member, where would the body be?" (1 Cor. 12:19). He goes on to say, "If one member suffers, all suffer together with it; if one member is honoured, all rejoice together" (verse 26). I dare add, "and if one member is shamed, we are all shamed." The Setswana saying; "*matlo go sha mabapi*," that is, huts environing each other burn together, is in concert with Paul's metaphor. One can never be sick alone. Again, in line with Paul's metaphoric representation, in Setswana one is often called *Kala'aka* (my branch), denoting this connectedness and relationality, indeed this "inescapable network of mutuality," without which we can neither know God nor worship the same.

Jesus, Motho per Excellence: A Reflection on Matthew 25:31-46

The historical Jesus, I would like to propose, was *Motho* per excellence. What made Him different, therefore, was the measure of the *Botho* dose he had. What we have in small doses, he had in the ideal dose. He had the ideal measure of *Botho* as God had intended us to have. *Botho*, one can therefore argue, is what Friedrich Schleiermacher referred to as God-consciousness, which he argues Jesus had in abundance. In *Botho*, we meet the very image of God, for *Botho* is *Bomodimo*. One with *Botho* has *Bomodimo*: Godness. Jesus' *Botho* is therefore the very *Imago Dei* we should strive to attain and reclaim. In him, we see one connected to those whom, because of our fallenness, we reject, shame, and treat with contempt: those we have shamelessly forced to reside in the margins of our societies.

In this context, Jesus identifies with those who are shamed. In fact, he does more than identify with them. He owns their situations; what is done to one is done **not for him** but **to him**. Our action or lack of action towards the hungry, naked, stranger, thirsty, imprisoned, and sick defines our relationship with Christ; here Jesus calls to mind the "I am because we are!" We are again reminded that our definition as *Batho* depends on our ability or inability to relate. When we do not act accordingly by meeting the needs of the needy, we do not only fail to carry our Christian obligation, we also fail to do our duties to the one we profess to believe in and serve. A poem by Canaan Banana captures the unfortunate contemporary Christian reality:

> ### Hungry, Lonely and Cold
> *When I was lonely,*
> *You left me alone.*
> *When I was homeless,*
> *You preached to me about*
> *the shelter of God's love.*
>
> *When I was hungry,*
> *You formed a humanity's*
> *club and discussed my hunger,*
> *When I was naked,*
> *You debated about the*
> *morality of my nakedness.*
> *When I was in prison,*
> *You guiltily crept into a*
> *cellar and prayed for my release.*

(Banana, 1981:21-22).

The above poem is a critique of Christian treatment of those in need of intervention. Often, we preoccupy ourselves with judging those in need than in helping them. The desire to go to heaven has made salvation so much of an individual enterprise that many Christians would rather focus on saving their skins and bask in self-assured individualistic hope to stroll through the pearly gates on the way to claiming their well deserved golden crown. Consequently, Christians have become too heavenly-minded to be of any real use. In so becoming, we have lost our core-business: as the salt and the light of the world, the saltiness and the light are lost! It is for the same reason that Jesus sentences such to damnation. The poem concludes by saying that when the subject was sick somebody was grateful to God for their own health. The poem went on to point out that the person appeared to be very holy and close to God and yet their neighbour still lacked food, was lonely and cold.

Jesus, in this context, is no more concerned with the morality of nakedness, sickness, hunger, imprisonment, and thirst, as he is about the necessary intervention. It is not important why he is or was in prison. He might be in there for doing something terrible to one of the family members but since *Botho* demands communalism, and as *Botho* falls apart at the rejection of one, the challenge is to embrace even those who violate the communal ethical codes. We can never even be excused from the "inescapable network of mutuality" by the mere fact that someone else has broken the relational code. To reject such would be to violate the *Botho* code. In the same way, for Christ it is not important what one suffers from, or how they contacted the disease, but that they are sick and ought to be embraced, loved, and cared for, and not judged. While we shame the HIV infected and sick, Jesus says, "I was HIV positive, with full blown AIDS, and you debated the morality of my status, judged me for having called the sickness and death upon myself!" Or better still, he puts it into the present tense: "I am HIV positive and you are busy debating the morality of my sickness!"

The life of Jesus was a life of the shamed, and it continues to be through those we shame in our everyday lives. What does this especially mean for the church? If "the least of these" are the family of Jesus, where does this leave the rest of those of us who are not on the margins? Indeed, there seems to be only one way for all of us to belong, that is, to be community, to be *communitas*, and therefore to be that which translates to having *Botho*. The challenge to humanity is to become a *koinonia* that is full of *splanchnizomai*: we need to be a community that is violently moved in our bowels to action for the good of those shamed and pained. Our *Seriti*, our magnetic field, ought to propel us to action, to draw near not to reject! In so doing, we become one with those in need, instead of being mere sympathizers. Through the needy, our relational God reveals to us the need we have to serve the Godself by serving the needy out of their needy situations. Jesus calls us to relate, which is to love in an active way.

Bringing Healing Where There is no Cure

Currently, there is no cure for HIV&AIDS. What we currently are struggling with is avoiding contacting or spreading the virus, and providing anti-retroviral drugs for those already affected. It is this absence of a cure that drives people to viewing HIV&AIDS as a moral instead of viral disease. It is because of this scenario that those infected are treated with contempt no person deserves. It is indeed this very situation that brings about a test most of us fail: a test to relate and love irrespective of one's circumstances!

I contend that many infected people do not die of the virus, but that instead they are murdered by the sin of human self-righteousness and self-preservation. We tend to place an unbearable load of blame and rejection on those we need to embrace more. Our lust for self-preservation drives us to the paranoia of even not wanting to touch the utensils of those known to be infected. We even deny them the healing touch they need so much.

Whereas there is yet no cure, there is nonetheless healing. *Botho* brings about healing. When one is welcomed and embraced, one feels part of. Like I mentioned earlier, we all need to be touched, because there is healing in it. The spiritual connection, the *seriti* that draws us together is activated when we do what we are commanded to do, that is to love God by loving those around us. Those infected are always advised to avoid stressful situations, but unfortunately one may not avoid being stigmatized and rejected, which are worse than the stressful situation to be avoided. *Botho* calls us to the very reality that we are all wounded, that we are all affected. It is only through approaching our reality as wounded healers that we would bring healing where there is no cure. The human touch and the human spirit have the capacity to effect healing; all we need to do is to invoke the spirit of connectedness in us to effect healing. The miracle of a touch and the spirit of connectedness, even more than anti-retroviral drugs can help those infected to live a more meaningful life. Consequently, this would bring about healing and wholeness to the wider *communitas.*

Theology, HIV&AIDS, and the Danger and Challenge of Gendering God

Often, people act out what they confess. There is power not only in the spoken but also in the written word. The Setswana saying goes, *"lefoko ga le boe, go boa monwana,"* that is, once a word is uttered there is no way of retrieving it; but as for a finger, the act of pointing it at one, in either an offending or an accusing way, can be reversed.

The challenge of teachers of theology is to take gender language seriously. Students of theology must be helped to use gender-sensitive language. It is easy to say there is no problem referring to God as "he." I would submit that language is paramount to the psychological construction of character. More often than not, we practice what we say, or have internalized. That is in fact why confession, for instance confessing "Christ as Lord" is so important for the Christian Church. St. Paul writes that confessing Jesus as Lord is a condition for salvation (Romans 10:9). Rather than using "He" or even "She" for God, for instance, one could use "Godself".

In Setswana, like in many African languages, we do not have such gender insensitive pronoun problems. We would say, "*O lorato*," while the English would have no gender-neutral pronoun to use there, hence the male pronoun "**He** is love." Maybe we could contribute to the expansion and development of theological language by using "O" wherever there is a need to use a pronoun for God. This will sound odd at the beginning, but imagine reading a book by an American or English five years from now, and you read: "O has called us to being, for O is love!" How exciting! Often, when one comes with such challenges, some laws of grammar are evoked as though they are not person-made and are therefore unalterable.

I must admit that due to the English language, and the idiom inherited from the missionary teachings, even behind the non-gendered "O" there is an invisible and inaudible gendered "**He!**" How many, times for instance, would one call God "*Modimo Ntate*" in one sentence while praying?

Gender: a Theological Construct

What do we think of when we think God? What do we see when we look at God through the eyes of our minds? As a child, I thought of God as a big, or rather fat old man with a long white beard who sits lazily on some kind of a throne. Is this not the picture the Book of Revelation suggests? A God sitting on a throne with the son Jesus sitting on his right hand? A kind of **male throne** is implied, complete with a male heir. Reflecting upon their salvation history, the children of Israel posit a warrior God who fights and wins wars for them. I cannot help but be reminded of a song by one Botswana gospel music artist, Juda Bosa, who sings, "Jehovah is the man of war, Jehovah mighty God, oh such a conqueror, Jehovah, mighty one!" If the divine is male, or should I put it the other way: if male is divine, mighty and glorious, what implications does this have on the non-male, and the treatment they receive?

While I agree that gender is a social construct, I tend to be getting more convinced that it is more of a Western theological construct. Listening to many call-in programmes over Radio

Botswana, it is the Bible, not Setwana culture, which is appealed to in justifying issues of gender inequality. Of course, one might argue that the Bible is used to affirm what people have always believed from their cultural standpoint. Turning to the Bible itself, and the reading of the same, is always a temptation for biblical critics to run to the defence of the Biblical writers, especially where the Bible seems to be oppressive. Instead of approaching or reading with a hermeneutic of suspicion, suspicion, even of our own hermeneutic, we approach the text as those who know exactly what the writers intended, which is, they actually are not saying what they seem to be saying. We approach it as if it is one of those familiar pieces of literature, whereas it is removed from our world in terms of context, time, and even worldview. The moment the Bible seems very familiar, be warned, you are off the mark!

The Bible and many other religious books have influenced peoples of the world, changing and affirming their worldviews to such an extent that their influence becomes the voice of orthodoxy. It is in this regard that even culture is at times not viewed at least as a voice of heterodoxy, but a complete antithesis of the normative, which maybe Christian, or whatever other faith, or better still, theological perspective. The Bible, I would propose, is but one of the numerous Godstories. The bible, like its reader is not devoid of meaning, which is also a product of the culture of the writers. It is in this regard that there is need to consider the importance of culture and one of the many important hermeneutical keys to unlock the meaning/meanings thereof. Furthermore, it is important not to approach any religious book, let alone theology from an absolutist, or ultra-conservative point of view.

In Setswana, or better still, in *Botho*, which is a non-Western theological approach, and indeed a non-literary yet authoritative text, more non-gendered names are used for God. God is called: *Kobontekana* (a blanket that covers all), *Seokama-ditshaba* (that which is above and covers all nations), *Moriti-o-tsididi-molapolosa balapi* (a cool/cold shade that gives rest to the weary), *Atladimaroba* (one with porous hands, denoting generousity),

Tintibane (a God by whom Batswana swear), *Morata-re-tshela yo o molemo* (the good one who wills us to live), *Timpa-kgolo* (big-bellied one, denoting wealth and abundance). Again God is referred to as *Kgosi*. In Setswana, *Kgosi*, though most of the times male, is referred to as *Mmabatho* or *Mmaarona* (mother of the people), and *Montle-poo* (a beautiful bull), a fusion of both feminine and masculine attributes.

Towards Exorcising the Demon of "Non-Male Subjugation"

To deal with the problem of negative gendering, which manifests itself in the subjugation of the women and girl-child making them more susceptible to HIV&AIDS infection; we need to deal with gendering God. I wonder if we can glorify the male without reversing the process on the non-male. For there to be any therapy, there is an unqualified need not only to identify, but more importantly, to confess and acknowledge the problem. The man possessed by demons named the demons; he called them legions. It was on the strength of naming them that he was healed. I would like to propose that the non-gendered names of God mentioned earlier are necessary in our exorcising of the demon at hand, as I am convinced that we can trace the subjugation of the non-male to our gendered perception of the divine. I must hasten to point out that I am in no way trying to imply that the Setswana culture is untainted, or free of the demon we need to exorcise. What I am suggesting is that we need to dig from the wells of *Botho* for names and metaphors that are necessary to carry out the near impossible task. I would like us to explore the **"girl-mother"** metaphor.

It is "ear-defying" for one to insult a female by pronouncing names of female genitalia in the Setswana tradition. On the other hand, it is not eyebrow-raising to hear the same with regard to males. Goats and cattle are rebuked using male genitalia insults, but it is a taboo to do the same using female genitalia insults. *Botho* mitigates this, as one is always reminded: "*Motho yoo mmaago yoo*," that is, "that person is your mother!" One's age here is never an issue. As said earlier, *Botho* is spiritual, and therefore a theological concept.

In this regard, this view of a female as a mother is important in shaping the mindset of theological students, especially in combating the gender inequalities that lead to the abuse of females to such an extent that they are viewed and treated as objects of male satisfaction and exploitation.

One story comes to mind here. A story is told of a young abusive husband who would always physically abuse his wife. Whenever the wife complains, she would be reminded: "women are donkeys!" One day, as they were driving, both in the best of moods, the husband, who was driving was not concentrating on the road. Suddenly, upon seeing a donkey on the road his wife screamed: "mind my mother in law!" As expected, the husband was not pleased that a donkey could be referred to as his very mother! As he fumed, the wife reminded him that women are donkeys!

Could it be a mere accident of history, confessional, or otherwise that Mary is referred to as *Theotokos,* the bearer of God? That she is referred to as the mother of God, while the same is not accorded to Joseph that Churches, especially the Roman Catholic Church, continues to revere Mary to such an extent that they are erroneously accused of worshipping her? Indeed, as *Botho* teaches, a female is a mother, to such an extent that she can be referred to as mother of God, a thing that could have been seen to be most blasphemous!

The girl-child and HIV&AIDS
Batho lebang kwa nokeng le utlwe
Letlametlo le sheleketlisa kwena
Letlametlo le roga kwena marete
Bogologolo di ne di sa rogane.

We need to be reminded here that regardless of age, "she is your mother!" The girl-child is at serious risk; she is in fact a threatened species. The implication of this is that humanity is a threatened species. The subjugation and abuse of the girl-child is tantamount to self-directed abuse and extermination. After all, I am because we are! It is in fact the abuse of the very image of God. *Botho*, as said, is the image of God; it is something of God in us. *Botho* dictates that people should live harmoniously with one another regardless of sex. It demands especially that males treat females as their own mothers. The spiritual connectedness that is inherent in *Batho* demands that we should see God in others, and again, that we should come to the realization that how we treat others does not define the recipient of the treatment; instead, it defines one meting out the treatment.

The moral fibre of our society is being corroded, and we qualify to be called *bo Bothoboile* (*Botho* has gone!). This scenario was long foreseen and foretold by our social prophets. The song quoted above, which was popularized by George Swabi, is a critique of such a situation. What is the moral of this song? Often we do not get to put on our hermeneutical antennas when such songs are heard. The language used often distracts us, and we consequently focus on the morality of the content, as in the words used and not the idiom, thereby ignoring the very moral that the singer intends to communicate. Worse still, some of our ultra-conservative Christian brothers and sisters would not even want to listen to such songs, as they allegedly "do not bring glory to God." Needless to say, such language, like that of the apocalyptic writings is meant to exclude those without an ear to hear what the spirit says to *Batho*. Let us take our hermeneutic tools and dissect this song; *Letlametlo* is a very small thing, a frog that has no business insulting and tossing *Kwena* around. All *Kwena* (crocodile) needs to do is open its big mouth and it would not even get the taste of what is in its mouth; *letlametlo* will simply be history! The question is why are they now quarrelling? Where does a frog get the guts to insult the crocodile?

As we deal with issues of HIV&AIDS, one of the most disturbing problems is inter-generational sexual relationships. This is even scarier as numbers of orphaned girl-children grow. Phrases like "*ke monnye ngwanaka*" (I am young my child) are not hard to come by nowadays. The reason *Letlametlo le sheleketlisa kwena* is because *kwena* has relegated itself to the status of the former. In this regard, the elderly men relate in an unorthodox manner with young girls by engaging in intergenerational sex. Now that the young girl knows and plays with *Kwena's* (elder men's) basic element, she finds it amusing and not wrong to name *(marete*-male genitalia) what she knows. It must be noted that in Setswana it is offensive to call out the other person's genitalia, especially if it is of the opposite sex. To name or call out the genitalia of an elderly person even is an abomination. Intergenerational sexual relationships point to the moral decadence where the *Botho* fibre is corroded. The song has a sense of nostalgia, the singer looks back to the time when both children and elders had *Botho*. These were times when the elderly respected themselves and got the same respect from the children in the spirit of *susu ilela suswana gore suswana a go ilele,* that is the elderly are supposed to observe taboos concerning their relating to the young so that the young ones could do the same. *Botho* calls for mutual respect and reciprocity.

The consequences of the above scenario are too numerous to mention, some of which are:

1. The spread of the virus reaches even those who are supposed to be our window of hope. The elderly, because of their economic power, take advantage of the less fortunate immature girl-children for their sexual exploits.
2. The virus is then spread among the younger generation thus exacerbating the problem.
3. The poor status of the young generation is perpetuated as they are turned into helpless dependents.
4. Loss of respect and *Botho* captured in *Letlametlo* insulting *Kwena*, and finally we are caught in a seemingly inescapable vicious cycle!

The Mother: a Caregiver

Discrimination and subjugation of both the girl-child and the womenfolk is detrimental to the whole society. The female is a mother because "*mmangwana o tshwara thipa ka fa bogaleng*", that is, the mother holds the knife by the blade in defence of her child. During these difficult times of HIV&AIDS, our survival rests in the hands of the "mothers." Our very survival therefore depends on how we treat them. "Mothers" are caregivers. In our society, as in many others, it is the women who care and nurse us, not only when we were children, but also continue to do so even when we are grown-ups, especially when we are sick. When the mother is not around, it is always the girl-child in the family who assumes the role of caregiver.

The infection of "some parents by HIV&AIDS forces" many girl-children to take care of their parents. After being orphaned, it is the girl-child who prematurely takes up the role of a mother. It is the girl-child who cares for and nurses other orphaned siblings. It is in this regard that we need to revisit our attitude towards the female folks to such an extent that we embrace the Setswana metaphor of a girl-child being a mother, irrespective of age.

Confronting the Challenges of Poverty

A few years down the time line, there was an uproar when President Mbeki of South Africa associated HIV&AIDS with poverty. Reality, however, shows that poor people are the most affected. In the so-called affluent countries, it is the poor, especially the non-whites who are hard hit. This calls to question the blessedness of the poor, or the saying that we will always have the poor amongst us. This further calls for a theology, and indeed a hermeneutic that mitigates ultra conservative Biblicism that is sponsored especially by American Tele-evangelism. To continue to look to the West with their affluence, for spiritual direction is to embrace the thinking of some of them, that they are chosen bearers of God's truth of salvation. It is to provide fodder for the thinking that power and wealth are signs of righteousness and God's favour. The danger here is that the West, which controls the world's economy, will continue to dictate how we should hear and experience God. The God we will hear and experience here is one who does not speak in our idiom, one who does not dance to the African rhythm.

To hear God anew, theological educators need to dig deeper into the African soul. We need to look inside, and turn the pages of our non-textual African Godstory text. In this text, we "read" about *letsema, molaletsa* and *mafisa*, among many others. Like in the early Church *communitas* (*koinonia*), where people lived together in an egalitarian commensality, sharing and doing things in common (*koina*) and for the common good of all (Act 2:42-47), *Botho* provided the same *koinonia.*.

Botho provides a safety net for the individual, especially the so-called have-nots. Among the Sotho-Tswana, there is a system of *mafisa* or cattle loaning. Those who have more cattle loan some to the poor. They are to look after them as they would of their own; they milk and use them for draught power, especially for ploughing, but cannot slaughter them. Those who work as herdsmen *go* through *tshwaelwa*, that is to be periodically given a heifer (Schapera, 1939:217). They are rewarded in this way as a means of paying, or rather thanking them for their assistance such that as soon as they have enough of their own, they move on to start their own cattle posts.

The other important system is that of *letsema/molaletsa* or work parties. For instance, if one needs to build a house or clear bushes and trees from a field, they would make some traditional brew, kill a goat or cow and invite others to work, sing, and feast at no cost. Schapera unfortunately mistakes the feasting part for payment (Schapera, 1939:255). In fact, eating together is an important activity that shows harmony and unity. In *Botho*, an individual "is never alienated from himself, for alienation occurs chiefly where individualism is the formula" (Simon, 1993:95). It is unfortunately true that the above have been either lost, or is being relegated to antiquity. We need to learn from these and adapt them to our contemporary situations. These are our stories of a few fish and bread feeding multitudes from our non-literary *Botho* text, which theological education should never shy from referring to.

Stigma and Poverty

That there are still those in multiple jeopardy (HIV&AIDS, stigma, discrimination, and poverty) points to inequitable distribution of resources. It points to the erosion of our spirituality. We are often reminded that "*molomo o'ja o roga o mongwe*" (when a mouth eats alone, it insults others), that "*bana ba motho ba kgaogana tlhogwana ya ntsi!*" (siblings share the head of a fly). The task of theological education is to challenge all that deface our being. We are a people of the hearth, where food and the warmth of being are shared even with those otherwise called strangers. The HIV pandemic demands that we consider, not with sympathy alone, but with compassion the needs of the affected and infected. With so many young adults dying and leaving behind orphans, the situation calls for "love-intervention." We need to consider, as a matter of gospel imperative, that these orphans, and those infected are the very brothers and sisters of Jesus. We need to be reminded again and again that whatever we do, by commission or omission, to the least of these, we do it to Jesus. The Lord requires of us "to do justice, and to love kindness and to walk humbly with God" (Micah 6:8). This God-walk is never a lonesome walk, it is a communal walk, and it demands that we walk with the afflicted, with the shamed and despised. The God-walk is a soothing and healing walk, a walk that heals where there is no cure! We therefore need to be reminded and warned that if we are not walking in the same direction as those who are the brothers and sisters of Jesus, we are walking in the wrong direction!

It is the obligation of theological educators to bring forth the Godstories of God's peoples everywhere, as witness for generations to see how their matriarchs and patriarchs have journeyed with God as they "penned" their Godstory. Our challenge is not only to challenge those who sit in the corridors of power to distribute the national cake equitably but more importantly to learn how our traditional Godstories counselled us to do so. Often when politicians and theologians consider fighting poverty, the focus turns to the governments and their countries' economies. Governments are often bashed for inequitable distribution of wealth. While this is part of both a political mandate and a prophetic imperative, it is important to consider what we can do to alleviate, if not to eradicate the problem. When faced with the hungry, Jesus often asked the disciples, "What do you have?" We have the means to effect change, to start the journey towards justice and healing by taking the first single step. Furthermore, the task of theological teachers is to move theology from being a mere academic theoretical undertaking, from being informational to being formational, from orthodoxy to orthopraxis.

We are often pricked and reminded by our Sages: "*se tshege yo o oleng mareledi a sa le pele*" (do not laugh at one who has fallen as the path is slippery further on), and "*se tshege tshege di ija mma motho di tla ja mmaago re tlaa go tshega*" (do not laugh when they eat somebody else's mother, we will laugh when they eat your mother). Furthermore, we are often instructed that "*fifing go tshwaranwa ka dikobo,*" that is when days are dark we must draw closer to each other. It is during the trying times of others, when they are inflicted, that we need to come closer together and see our being clearly being defined by how we treat them in times of great need.

Conclusion

Weep not, child
Weep not, my darling
With these kisses let me remove your tears,
The ravening clouds shall not be long
victorious,
They shall not long possess the sky [...]
Walt Whitman

The Godstory is an unfinished story. It has not been concluded in the bible. Our theology, while guided and dependent on "Holy Books" should not be blind to other "Holy non-literary texts." In fact, it is these texts that can help us understand the written text. More importantly, they can help us know who we are and what makes us, that it is in caring in the *Botho* way, which is the divine way, and that we can relate and participate in the perichoretic relationality. In *Botho*, through music, poetry, stories, mythology, and sagacity, we see and hear God speak, act, and relate through our human history.

In it we not only have what we need to complement the literary text captured in the Bible, but instead we have what is fundamental to understanding what is written in the Bible.

I am therefore in concert with Bowley who introduces the word "anthology" and suggests it "is a picturesque and accurate term for the Bible." Anthology is from the Greek words (*anthos* and *logos*) that together mean a bouquet or a gathering together of flowers. Hence, the Bible is "a beautiful bouquet of diverse literary creation" which "communities of faith have arranged differently, sometimes discarding, sometimes adding, sometimes putting into the background what another places in prominent position" (Bowley, 1999:11). In line with my earlier proposal, I would further suggest, as a bouquet, the Bible; is not all that flowers are. It is a bouquet that, being made of flowers, is not made out of all the flowers that can make a bouquet.

The Bible, I would suggest further, is not the ultimate bouquet, but that it is one among other bouquets and flowers that make up the ultimate, which is "The God-story" that completes the aesthetic landscape of religious faith. As such, the Bible is but one among many texts, written and oral (itself a product of oral texts), explicit and implicit, that together can tell the God-story. The Bible cannot be the whole story, because God and God's perichoretic relationality cannot be fully reduced, captured, and articulated in any literary text, no matter how voluminous.

It is in this regard that Bowley (1999:9) argues that for moderns to jump to the conclusion, whenever they hear "*torah*" or divine "word" in the bible that it refers to the written law is to "underestimate the value of orality in ancient Israel." The Bible can therefore be viewed as a microcosmic representation of the macrocosmic reality of God's perichoretic relationality with humanity and created order. It can only be through the reading of the bible and listening to other stories of peoples' experiences of and with God that God can dance to the local and particular rhythmic and harmonic patterns and arrangements of all peoples, with their musical improvisations and spontaneous creativity that define and colour their musical landscape.

There is a need to read the Bible and other "Holy Books" in a liberating way. As inferred earlier, literalism and inerrancy approaches are more detrimental than liberating. they have imprisoned and subjugated the poor, and especially the women. It is not a mere accident of history and creation that females are the ones who are more affected by poverty, diseases, abuse, and all unpleasant things in life. *Botho* is what constitutes God's image in us, and that, which is divine, knows not what is male or female.

The main theological task is, therefore, to unravel the mystery of *Botho* as divine; of *Motho* understood as divine. It is to wrestle with the notion that according to the *Botho* worldview, one can never be a Christian or attain salvation *a se na Botho* (without *Botho*). This, in view of the HIV&AIDS pandemic means without the HIV positive, we cannot attain salvation. That we in fact need "them" more than we think they need "us." How we relate to, treat by commission or omission those infected defines not them but us. It takes *Motho* to worship God, it takes *Botho* for "one" to be *Motho*. Consequently, those without *Botho* are not *batho* and cannot worship God. *Botho*, as earlier said, is the very *Imago Dei* we possess; it is that very divinity Jesus had in abundance. With *Botho*, there is hope for the afflicted, hope that "the ravening clouds shall not be long victorious; that they shall not long possess the sky [...]."

References

Banana, C. (1981). *The Gospel According To The Ghetto*. Gweru: Mambo Press.

Booth, N. S. Jr. (1977). The View from Kasongo Niembo. In Newell S.

Booth, Jr. ed. *African Religions: A Symposium*. New York: NOK Publishers, Ltd.

Bowley, (ed.) (1999). *Living Traditions of the Bible*. St. Louis: Chalice Press.

James E. B. (1999). A Library of Tradition: The Beginnings of the Bible. In:

James E. Bowley (ed.) *Living Traditions of the Bible*. St. Louis: Chalice Press.

Ford, D. F. (1999). *Theology: A Very Short Introduction*. New York: Oxford University Press.

Hick, J. (1976). *Death and Eternal Life*. London: Macmillan Press.

King, N. Q. (1970). Religions *of Africa: A Pilgrimage Into Traditional Religions*. New York: Harper & Row.

Macquarrie, John.1977 *Principles of Christian Theology*. London: SCM Press Ltd.

Mbiti, J. (2000). *African Religions and Philosophy*. Bloomington: University of Indiana Press..

Ray, B. C. (1970). *African Religions: Symbol, Ritual, and Community*. New Jersey: Prentice Hall

Schapera, Isaac. *A Handbook of Tswana Law and Custom*. London: Oxford University Press, 1939.

Setiloane, G. M (1986). *African Theology: An Introduction*. Johannesburg: Skotaville Publishers.

Simon, B. (1993). *Death and the Invisible Powers*. Bloomington: University of Indiana Press.

Suchocki, Marjorie Hewitt. *God Christ Church: A Practical Guide to Process Theology*. New York: Crossroads, 1989.

Tillich, P. (1967). *Systematic theology: Three volumes in one*. Chicago: The University of Chicago Press.

Washington, J. M. (ed.) (1986). *A Testament of Hope: The Essential Writings and Speeches of Martin Luther King, Jr.* New York: Harper Collins Publishers.

The Concept of Botho and HIV&AIDS in Botswana

CHAPTER TWO

The Setswana Concept of *Botho*
Unpacking the Metaphysical and Moral Aspects

Joseph B. R. Gaie

Introduction

The word *Botho* is a noun of classes 1.2 (one two) and 14 (fourteen) in the Setswana language (Mogapi, 1984:12). It comes from the root *–tho* (Mogapi, 1984:20). The word means "a human being" as a metaphysical entity, and "a person" at a moral level. These concepts will be examined below for us to understand the moral significance of this term in this book.

This chapter argues that the term "*Botho*" has metaphysical and ethical aspects. At a metaphysical level, *Botho* denotes some reality with an ontological status. It denotes the existence or presence of a specific or specifiable being. In other words, the term can be understood to reflect the "whatness" of something—that which makes the thing itself. The Setswana tradition has a way in which it understands what a *Motho* is.

What a *Motho* is, or whatever *Botho* has is morally important. In fact, *Botho* defines morality. This term is therefore not just a metaphysical term. It has moral importance that needs to be understood if one has to meaningfully discourse about the traditional thinking of Batswana, and to some extent, African traditional thought. So, in order to explicate this more the chapter deals with the metaphysical elements of *Botho*, the importance of the metaphysical elements of the term, and the moral elements of *Botho*.

The Metaphysical Elements of *Botho*

At this level, we are looking at being—that is, what makes *Botho*. We want the essence of *Botho* such that we would say that the absence of that thing in a being would disqualify it from being called a *Motho*. In Setswana, *Botho* is simply humanbeinghood, or the essence of being a human person. It is that which separates people or human beings from any other animal species. At a metaphysical level, there is a thing that has the essence of *Botho* or humanbeinghood. The question then is what a *Motho* is. Kwasi Wiredu (1991:31) has provided something close to the answer. According to him, a human person is that which is born of communication, a product of culture. It includes the mind, and an ability or power to conceptualize and articulate. This power is usually realizable in an evolutionary process of cultural socialization. This means a *Motho* is both physical/biological and immaterial—the mind. A *Motho*, or,

> being a human person implies having the capacity for reflective perception, abstraction, and inference. In their basic nature these mental capacities are the same for all humans irrespective of whether they inhabit Europe, Asia or Africa, just as in their basic nature the instinctive reactions of, say, the frogs of Europe are the same as those of the frogs of Africa. [...] there is a common human identity (Wiredu, 1991:32-33).

Lesiba *et. al.* agree as they argue that:

Although there are differences with reference to the constituting parts of a person, there is agreement that the person consists basically of a material aspect and a 'spiritual' aspect or aspects. We thus have a dualism with the resulting question of how these different aspects function together (1991:146).

In the case of Setswana a *Motho* can be described materially and spiritually, morally and epistemologically. At a material or physical level, the *Batswana* refer to *Motho* as *"ke motho yo moleele"* (he or she is a tall person). They will also refer to a corpse as *Motho*. Talking of the corpse, for example, they usually report back to those who remained at home when a member of the family was going to be buried, and say, *"re mmolokile"* (we have buried him or her). This is a clear reference to the corpse as a person. Another example is that Batswana believe that when the corpse of a person is in the house, or at home, there should never be noise in order to respect the dead person. They will say that *"o mo ntlong"* (he or she is in the house).

The spiritual nature or aspect of a person in the Setswana tradition is also reflected in the way Batswana talk about death. All living things are said to *"swa"* or die, including human beings. It is also very clear that the death of a person is referred to in a peculiar way. Batswana do no usually say *motho o sule* (dead), even though they can say that. They usually say *"o tsamaile/ile"* (he or she has gone); *o re tlogetse* (he or she has left us); *o tlhokafetse* (he or she is missing or cannot be found*); ga a yo* or *ga a sa tlhole a le teng* (he or she is not or no longer there).

We shall talk about the moral aspect of *Botho* below, so the next issue to talk about here is the epistemological aspect of *Motho*. To say that a *Motho* is epistemological in Setswana tradition means that knowledge is part of the definition of what a *Motho* is. It is an aspect of the essence of a person. Batswana usually say that *"motho ke phologolo e e botlhale go feta diphologolo tsotlhe,"* (the most intelligent animal is a human being). The word *botlhale* means wisdom, intelligence, being clever, and cunning. An intelligent and wise being is that which is able to conceptualize reason assuming the many laws of thought, such as the Principle of non contradiction—any proposition cannot be true when its negation is true (Not A and −A at the same time); Principle of identity—a thing is itself (A is A); and excluded middle or LEM (law of excluded middle) A is B or A is not B (P or −P). There is no middle ground where A will both be and not be B; and a whole is greater than any of its parts (Lacey, 1996:176). When a child has done something requiring intelligence only befitting a human being, Batswana say *"ke motho tota"* (he or she is a real human being). That means, being intelligent and knowledgeable shows the child as a real human being.

The Importance of the Metaphysical Concept of *Botho*

It is important to emphasize from the outset that the concept of *Botho* is morality itself. Just like any kind of essence at a metaphysical level, the essence of *Botho* is illusive in that it is difficult to define or pin down. There is nothing in particular that can easily be pointed out as the essence of *Botho*. On the other hand, it is generally accepted that certain behaviour traits reflect the nature and essence of *Botho*. This is not a big problem for the proponents of *Botho* as a viable philosophical and moral position, because morality itself has the same problem of pinning down what really makes something wrong. Sogolo (1993:126) has also made the same observation. In fact, some people have sought to solve the problem by suggesting that there is nothing which is wrong as such, only emotional attitudes towards certain things cause people to think there is something wrong (Popkin &Stroll, 1986:55; Gensler, 1998:58). Yet, others have suggested relativism as a solution—that the wrongness or rightness of actions vary from society to society, culture to culture, or person to person (Billington, 1988:35ff).

Rantao (May 2002), defines *Botho* as "good personality". He also brings out the important idea that in Setswana, a person who has no *Botho* is viewed as not being a *Motho* or person. When a person does things, which are viewed to be immoral or unbecoming, they are simply described as the negation of personhood—*ga se motho*—he is not a person. This negation of personhood is both metaphysical and ethical in that the definition of a person is that of a human being who has loyalties to his kin, country, and everybody else. Furthermore, according to Rantao, the Setswana tradition extols the virtue of love. It is this kind of metaphysical reality that gives rise to the moral person—society expects certain behaviour from the individual. These behaviours will reflect the metaphysical reality called *Motho*, as a being that captures the moral concept of *botho*.

To expound on the above, in the English language people can speak of an old car as not being a car. What this means is that even though the car has the essential elements of a car, there are some aspects of those essential elements of the car that are missing. This suggests degrees of being. There is a sense in which the car is not a car. This is analogous to *Motho*. For example, a *Motho* who is not a *Motho* is one who is morally deficient. What this means is that whereas a *Motho* is a being of a certain ontological status, there are statuses between *Botho* and non-*Botho* that we can talk about and which are important.

It is important to consider the metaphysical elements of *Botho* because it will help in understanding the concepts of *Botho-Motho*. A real or proper *Motho* is a being with essential elements that include rationality and morality. This is important in that the essential elements of *Motho* will enable us to understand what things the *Motho* as *Motho* should and should not do.

Modern critics of Setswana traditional outlook point out that in the modern day era of HIV and AIDS, cultural beliefs fuel the spread of the disease. For example, goes the argument, because the Setswana tradition encourages young people, especially girls, to be subservient to elders, unscrupulous elderly relatives impose themselves on young girls and end up sexually abusing them, thus exposing them to the dangers of HIV and AIDS. The youngsters do not resist because they are taught to obey the elders.

That could be what happens in practice, but then it would be indicative of either the abuse of Setswana tradition, or a misunderstanding of what really a *Motho* is. Since rationality, morality, and epistemology are essential elements of a *Motho*, it seems untenable to propose a Setswana culture that promotes the violation of Batswana youth. Taking for granted that abusing young girls is immoral, it appears to follow that Setswana tradition, which defines *Motho* as a moral being, or *Botho* as being moral, would not tolerate the abuse of children by elders. As a matter of historical fact, child molesters were severely punished. Child molesters, those who committed incest and homosexuals were among those people who were killed because it was believed that they were committing taboo acts—*botlhodi*.

So, we can say that a *Motho* and *Botho* define what ought and ought not be done. This shows the relevance of metaphysics to a good understanding of *Botho* and *Motho*. This is not any different from the Western tradition. Because I am a human being, I am not expected, in the moral sense, to do certain things such as cruelty to animals and human beings. The Setswana tradition dictates that because you are a *Motho* you cannot abuse children. Because you are a *Motho*, you cannot allow yourself to be abused by an elderly person. As noted above, rationality is part of the defining characteristics of a *Motho*. A clever child would know what to expect from the elders. For example, they cannot be cruel to the child and claim that it is dictated by culture. Of course, people can be quick to point out that Setswana traditionalists were very cruel, but that can hardly pass the test of truth, because there were always limits to what a person could do to others. The fact that some people abused their status does not invalidate the view that Setswana tradition defined *Motho* as a being that should not do certain things, including letting oneself to be abused and abusing others.

The traditional Setswana culture is very protective of children, because as suggested above, the acceptable activities of a being are defined by what it is. *Botho* defines that because people are what they are, they have to behave in a certain way towards children, also because of what children are. For example, there is a saying in Setswana, *e re o ntima, o mphele ngwana.* This can be translated to mean a few things. Firstly, if a person has something against his neighbour or fellow citizen, it does not mean he should take it on their children. People should rather treat their fellow citizens' children as if they do not have anything against their parents. Secondly, treating fellow human beings' children unkindly because they have something against their parents is the most selfish thing to do. Lastly, treating the children of people that somebody has something against well is equivalent to treating the people themselves well (Seboni, 1962:25). It is also critical here to note that for Batswana *ga go ke go twe o gola leng, go a twe o tsalwa leng* (literally meaning: it is never said "when are you going to grow up?" It is said, "when are you born?"). The saying means that once one is born, they are a *Motho*, or a person (Seboni, 1962: 30). This is important because it means a child has the same metaphysical status as an elderly person. This is consistent with Kaphagawani who has argued that for the Chewa in Malawi,

> It is indeed the case that elders tended to have an epistemological monopoly over the young. But to concede this point is not to assert an ontological distinction between the elders and the young; rather, it is merely to point out an epistemological difference; the young are not onotologically less human than the elders.
> (Kaphagawani, 1991:173).

The Moral Elements of *Botho*[1]

Botho, as stated above, is simply morality (Mmolai & Gaie, 2003; Gaie, 2005). To say that a person has *Botho* is the same as saying that they are morally good. To say they do not have *Botho* is the same as saying they are immoral. This position is not clearly articulated as one complete argument, but can be gleaned from various writings and utterances, some of which will be looked at below. In this section, it will become clear that *Botho* is the most important moral term that is used in Setswana. I will also point out that it is related to the Zulu or Ndebele term *"ubuntu"*. It is

---

[1]The questions of whether or not Africans and by extension, Batswana have a traditional philosophy and a morality that are comparable to other systems such as Europe are taken for granted. We hold the view that Setswana traditional thinking is universalizable to the same extent and with similar difficulties to European cultures. So we are not going to have that debate here. Godwin Sogolo (1993: 119ff) for example, has ably demonstrated this position.

sometimes used loosely, but mostly it is moral in content wherever and whenever it is used.

Ubuntu

One concept that has been expressed in the literature is *Ubuntu*. This concept, in my view, should be understood synonymously with *botho*. It is simply a Zulu/Ndebele Xhosa variant of the same concept. **Ubuntu** expresses the essence of *Botho*. It is the treatment of people as persons deserving special moral consideration. *Ubuntu*, in other words, is the morality of the African whereby the Africans see themselves as being what they are because of people. *Ubuntu* is "true humaneness" (Prinsloo, 1991:42). *Botho* or *Ubuntu* is the way of life in which rationality and morality are seen as foundations for community life. It is a way of viewing the universe as an environment within which the self-realization of an individual is only possible through and in others. This concept really means that there are certain things that cannot be done in this society given the importance of reason. For example, some people might think that traditional Setswana cultures gave room for child abuse. This is not possible, given the fact that Setswana traditional culture is rational. From the culture, it can never be *Botho* for an elderly person to abuse a child. In fact, incest is viewed as *botlhodi* (taboo), which could result in the abuser being killed. The idea of respect for elders does not mean the elders can abuse children without the latter objecting. But this is not true as sayings such as *susu ilela suswana gore suswana a tle a go ilele* (the elders should respect the young so that the young can respect them), precisely meaning that the elderly does not merit respect when he abuses children, and therefore they cannot accord him the respect that is accorded to elders. *Ubuntu* or *Botho* is also simply virtue as expressed in the Western tradition.

Understanding of Botho

The Mmegi newspaper (30th March 2004, p.7) carried an editorial entitled "we want PBRS with *Botho*". It explained that the performance-based reward system would be welcome in Botswana if it would involve the civil service becoming service-oriented, and the service done efficiently, courteously, and with all the kindness and good human relations possible. The civil service would stop being a terrorizing monster to the public, which ordinary people needing service would try to avoid as much as possible, and become a welcoming and humane one.

Botho *as virtue*

The Batswana have shown that they have the concept of *Botho* as virtue. This is shown in the case of taxi men who returned over P4million (about US$667 000) that they found on the road to the bank (Mmegi Monitor, 2002ab:6, 8; Geoflux, 2002:13; Maleke, 2002:6). The action of the taxi men was extolled as virtue. Monty Chiepe is quoted as having said:

> This is the highest demonstration of honesty and botho. What is even more touching about this is the fact that taxi men demonstrate this very important Setswana attribute, a group of people not considered the most probable for these virtues (botho and honesty). What makes their deed even more outstanding is the fact that it happens at a time when everybody seems to be preoccupied with materialism at the expense of values that make us Batswana. (Mmegi Monitor, 2002a: 6).

This view reflects Batswana as virtuous persons who ought to be rewarded for honesty. The view goes on to see *Botho* as what makes them who they are. Virtue is being someone who radiates *Botho*, someone capable of being trustworthy even when in a tempting situation. The action of the taxi men is described as what "reflects the true spirit and nature of our being as Batswana, or even further as Africans. Their actions touch right to the full definition of 'BOTHO'; '**Motho ke motho ka ba bangwe'**" (Geoflux, 2002:13). The statement translates into "a person is a person through, and because of other persons". Geoflux, a company in Botswana led by Mr Monty Chiepe, Botswana Society, a community of prominent Batswana, and Mmegi Monitor, a local newspaper felt that it was *botho*—morally desirable to ensure that people who have behaved virtuously are not ridiculed like it was happening to the taximen (Maleke, 2002:6), but they were to be honoured and encouraged. The news paper reported that the taxi men who returned the money that they found were vilified and ridiculed by some members of society accusing them of being fools who could not take advantage by keeping the money that they found lost on the road. As a country that believes in virtue, Botswana ought to protect virtue and encourage virtuous behaviour.

On the other hand, Botshelo complains about the fact that the said taxi men have attracted a lot of attention simply because they returned money to the bank. He points out that he appreciates the fact that they have behaved virtuously. He also points out that the security company that was supposed to guard the money did something consistent with *Botho*, as it gave the taxi men something. *Botho*, according to his understanding, means that virtuous people should be rewarded, and what is of paramount importance is not the size of the reward, but the meaning of the reward. He takes issue with the fact that the taxi men were capturing the headlines because the issue they were involved in was money, which is not as important as human life. Botshelo points out the fact that the media did not harp on the discovery of foetuses in Selibe Phikwe,[2] and the incident will soon be forgotten in spite of the fact that it is an issue of great importance. Botshelo is worried that the person who reported the presence of those foetuses ought to be seen as a hero who personifies *Botho*, but society does not seem to care very much about him. Botshelo agrees that *Botho* is virtue. He points out "Mrs Phumaphi, using her position and authority, was able to convince the *Ditsela tsa Itshetso Society* to donate one of its houses initially earmarked

---

[2]Selibe Phikwe is one of the towns in the central part of the country. One resident of the town discovered a hole filled with foetus' corpses, which led to the arrest and trial of a local traditional doctor who was accused of helping women to commit abortion.

for the homeless, to Boitumelo Morapedi to share with her child. This is *botho*" (Botshelo, 2002: 24).

Another example of *Botho* as virtue is seen in the case where the Botswana National Vision 2016 chairperson is quoted as having called upon the Church to spice their sermons with teachings about *Botho* as portrayed in the vision. The chairperson of the vision council, Dr. Gloria Somolekae, is said to have acknowledged the compliance between the teaching of the Church and Botswana's National Vision 2016. This is an apparent reference to the Christian teaching on virtue. Peter Hikhwa is quoted as having said that the Church is able to build people morally (Matshediso, 2004:4).

Lack of virtue is lack of *Botho*, and virtue is having *Botho*. S.M. Mosojane (2001:17) argues that in African traditions people do not criticize someone in mourning. They would rather wait for the mourning period to pass before they can take issue with the bereaved, if they think there is some issues to settle. He argues that in their village there is an individual who is insensitive enough to criticize someone, and falsely accuse them of misusing council property whilst the person they are attacking is mourning. This unwarranted attack is, in his view, lack of *botho*.

Mmegi, (2003:16) is concerned about the apparent "public indecency," evident during music festivals held purportedly to raise funds for HIV and AIDS reduction activities. The commentary lists a few examples of some activities that end up with people having sexual encounters in an unacceptable manner. This necessitates the need for national soul-searching, an introspection to find out if the Botswana nation has become too permissive. The commentary suggests an apparent lack of virtue in the nation of Botswana, or an equivalent of lacking *Botho*. Naledi (2003:2), a Setswana publication of Mmegi has also taken up the topic of *Botho* in its commentary. According to this commentary, it is a happy occasion to have witnessed the President of Botswana, F. Mogae and some eminent persons in society launching the special fund to honour all members of the nation who have shown *Botho* in a special way. It is of concern that the spirit of *Botho* has been waning in the nation of Botswana for some time. The hope is that it will be rekindled by the few acts of virtue that are encouraged by activities such as the fund to honour all members of the nation who have shown *Botho* in a special way. The commentary goes on to congratulate a group of men belonging to a recreational football club for standing against the abuse of women and children. It then urged them to cooperate with the Society of Men Against Aids (SMAA), so that the two can have a good social impact. The existence of these groups shows *Botho* as a national virtue. Mooketsi (2003:2) quotes Limit Nkala as having argued that rape is wrong because *Botho* demands consent. Rape as lacking virtue is simply lack of *Botho*.

T. Man (2003:16) has argued that *Botho* is important for the realization of a compassionate, loving, and caring nation. The nation can attain *Botho* if parents become role models for their children. In so doing, they will respect their children, show compassion to them, and they will not use "vitriolic language" when they talk to the children. Parents are supposed to uphold moral standards, but nowadays they are nothing but morally bankrupt by being rude, aggressive, and callous. They are "deficient of proper morals"; they commit "horrendous atrocities" to their children; there are "unprecedented and unparalleled cultural and moral disintegration"; defilement is on the increase with both women and men being perpetrators, and some men rape their daughters. "Such behaviour" he argues, "is totally disturbing and not inimical for the construction of a nation which values *Botho*". He concludes: "a nation without high standards of morality faces a bleak future".

Another example of *Botho* as virtue is reflected by Mmegi Monitor (2002a: 8), where the cultural traditions are seen as forming part of the virtuous status of the state. The commentary points out the fact that the way young people dress and speak nowadays gives some credence to fears that the nation is losing its soul. It also points out that people who accused virtuous members of society of being naïve and foolish when they returned millions of Pula they found on the road is a sign that *Botho* is gone. Nevertheless, the president should honour these gentlemen to show that theirs was "a noble act".

In another case of identifying *Botho* with virtue, Mmegi (2004b) argues that *Botho* demands good behaviour even when one feels betrayed. The comment was raised by the fact that the South African Football Association did not vote for Botswana's candidature in a CAF election, in spite of the fact that Batswana supported South Africa for a long time. The comment came just before the FIFA vote to determine the 2010 world cup host. People were divided as to whether the Botswana delegate to FIFA should vote against South Africa hosting the tournament, since the South Africans had "betrayed" Batswana earlier on during the CAF elections presidency. The commentary points out that Batswana are related to South Africans in a very special way. *Botho* demands that the former should help the latter, even if they have betrayed them before. Hence, the South Africans can learn what *Botho* is by being treated with *Botho*.

Conclusion

This chapter has argued for the understanding of *Botho* as a concept that has metaphysical, moral, and ethical elements. These elements need to be well understood if we are going to discourse meaningfully about the different moral issues of our society, including the HIV and AIDS pandemic. There is just no way that a person behaving in a way that is consistent with *Botho* can intentionally cause harm to another person. A misunderstanding of the term *Botho* can make some people think that behaving according to *Botho* can, for example, fuel the spread of HIV in the case of elders abusing the young, and hoping they do not resist them because it would be unlike *Botho* to do so.

References

Billington, R. (1988). *Living Philosophy. An Introduction to Moral Thought* (2nd ed.). London & New York: Routledge.

Botshelo, D.M. (2002). Botho campaign off the mark. In: *The Botswana Guardian*, Friday November 29, 2002, p.24.

Gaie, J.B.R. (2004). *The Ethics of Medical Involvement in Capital Punishment. A Philosophical Discussion*. Dordrecht & Boston: Kluwer Academic Press.

_____ (2005). "Social Responsibility of Corporations and Business ethics: The role of Moral Theory and Botho" BIAC Journal Vol. 2 No.1 May 2005, pp.40-65.

Geoflux (Pty) Ltd (2002). Let's Reward the two taximen for exemplary 'botho' action. In: *Mmegi Monitor* 29 October-14 November 2002, Vol.2 No. 42, p.13.

Gensler H.J. (1998). *Ethics. A contemporary introduction*. London: Routledge.

Lacey, A.R. (ed.) (1996). *A Dictionary of Philosophy* (3rd ed.). London & New York: Routledge.

Lesiba et. al. (1991). Metaphysical Thinking in Africa. In: Coetzee, P.H. &

Roux, A.P.J. (eds) *Philosophy from Africa. A Text with Readings*. Oxford: Oxford University Press., pp.134-148.

Maleke, L. (2002). Million-Pula Taximen Land in Trouble. In: *Mmegi Monitor,* 15-21 October 2002, Vol.2 No. 42, p.6.

Man, T. (2003). Botswana's morality is degenerative. In: *Mmegi*, Wednesday 17th December 2003, Vol. 20, N0. 82, p. 16.

Matshediso, T. (2004). Colour sermons with 'botho.' *The Midweek*, Sun Wednesday August 4 2004, p.4.

Mmegi, (2003). Alarming behaviour at music festivals. In: *Mmegi*, Wednesday 3rd December 2003, Vol. 20, N0. 74, p. 16.

Mmegi, (2004a). We want PBRS with Botho. In: *Mmegi*, Tuesday 30th March 2004, Vol. 21, N0. 49, page, 7.

Mmegi, (2004b). Give SA a lesson in Botho. In: *Mmegi*, Friday 14 May 2004, Vol. 21, N0. 75, page, 12.

Mmegi, (2004c). Our Moral Standards are Sinking. In: *Mmegi*, Wednesday 21 July 2004, Vol.21, No. 110, page, 6.

Mmegi Monitor (2002a). Where is Botho? In: *Mmegi Monitor*, 15-21 October 2002, Vol. 3 No. 40, p.8.

Mmegi Monitor (2002b). Help Beckons For Taximen. In: *Mmegi Monitor,* 22-28 October 2002, Vol. 3 No. 41, p.6.

Mmolai, S. & Gaie, J.B.R. (2003). "The Concept of Botho and Efforts to Combat HIV/AIDS": *Opportunity or Challenge?* Paper presented at the 6th Biennial National Council on Teacher Education Conference, Towards The Realisation of a Developed and Informed Nation: A Challenge for Educators, Gaborone.

Mogapi, K. (1984). *Thutapuo ya Setswana* (2nd ed.) Cape Town and Gaborone: Longman.

Mooketsi, L. (2003). Borre ba ganana le kgokgontsho. In: *Naledi*, 13-19 Seetebosigo 2003, p.1.

Mosojane, S.M. (2001). What happened to Botho? In: *The Botswana Guardian*, Friday August 10 2001, p.17.

Naledi, (2003). Botho. In: *Naledi*, 13-19 Seetebosigo 2003, p.2.

Popkin R.H. & Stroll, A. (1986). *Philosophy* (Revised Edition). Gaborone and London: MadeSimple Books, Heinemann Professional Publishing.

Prinsloo, E.D. (1991). Ubuntu culture and participatory management. In: Coetzee, P.H. & Roux, A.P.J. (eds) *Philosophy from Africa. A Text with Readings*. Oxford: Oxford University Press, pp.41-51.

Rantao, P. (2002). *The Role of manners in Tswana Culture—Boitshwaro mongwaong ya Setswana*. In: *The Botswana Gazette*, Wednesday 29 may 2002, p. E4.

Seboni, M.O.M. (1962). *Diane le Maele a Setswana*. Cape Town: Lovedale Press.

Sogolo, G. (1993). *Foundations of African Philosophy. A definitive Analysis of Conceptual Issues in African Thought*. Ibadan: Ibadan University Press.

Wiredu, K. (1991). Are there cultural universals? In: Coetzee, P.H. & Roux, A.P.J. (eds.) *Philosophy from Africa. A Text with Readings*. Oxford: Oxford University Press., pp.31-40.

The Concept of Botho and HIV&AIDS in Botswana

CHAPTER THREE

The Maid, *Botho*, and HIV&AIDS Infections: The Economic and Ethical Perspectives

Innocent S. Botshelo

Introduction

The continuingHIV&AIDS infection amongst Batswana is still a cause for concern. The search for reasons on the continuing new infections will therefore carry on. Perhaps one of the reasons could be the lack of *Botho* in our people. *Botho* is sometimes referred to as humanity; it is a phenomenon, a theory, or a framework that advocates for compassion and care amongst the human race. This chapter will look at ways in which the maid is disadvantaged economically, as compared to other workers.

It will use the *Botho* framework to show how failure to practice it indirectly, and sometimes directly, contributes to the HIV&AIDS pandemic not abetting. It will also look at the economic implications of the current practices and strategies adopted in the recruitment and employment of maids. These do not directly address the maids as a part of the solution to the HIV&AIDS pandemic, but serve to alert that in failing to practice *Botho*, we increase and contribute to the infection's incidences. The chapter will also attempt to respond to issues such as:

1. Do employers acknowledge housemaids and extend their
   gratitude to them in other ways beyond monetary rewards?
2. Who has the moral responsibility to change if necessary,
   and what is the morally acceptable way?

The moral aspect to these questions is whether there is a moral
justification for the *status quo* to prevail? Morality hinges around
positive attributes of humanity, compassion, care, and unconditional
love for others. Perhaps the notion of *Botho* needs to be rekindled
to stimulate positive attitudes that would fight negative pressures
and challenges.

In failing to extend *Botho* to the maid, do we not only risk
transferring infections to our neighbours and relatives, but also
compound the economic hardships to our fellow human beings and
their dependents. How correct is this statement?

Is Botho an Exogenous Economic Force?

Botho is generally extended by all people at all ages, and it does not
discriminate by colour, gender, wealth, status, or age. I would like to
see *Botho* as humanity, a mindset of individuals of a community
that cares and is compassionate to its people. When put into practice,
no conditions, benefits, or rewards are expected or attached to it;
Botho is therefore a virtue. This is fast diminishing as part of
Setswana culture.

In conducting a study on the economic impact of HIV&AIDS
infections amongst maids, I found that it would appear like people
have adopted individualistic behaviours that protect their income
earning capability. It was evident in the responses from participants
that HIV&AIDS infections are still a thorny issue. Respondents
indicated that they tend to make choices, and subsequently decisions
that are primarily influenced by economic or financial earnings or
gains.

Economic choices are about forgoing one thing in order to get
the other, and normally referred to as opportunity costs. Sometime,
the opportunity cost is intertwined with moral obligations, and in
some instances, the economic choice is more practical and thus

overrides the moral choice. It is therefore not surprising that both the employer and employee in the survey conducted did not want to address the issue of HIV&AIDS because of their fears.

Just like their maid, the employers face a dilemma of economic pressure of a different nature. The employer seeks the service of a housemaid because they have to keep a job, which in turn provides them the basic economic needs. Because good maids with the *Botho* quality are scarce, they are forced not to enquire about HIV&AIDS status. If they ask of the maid's HIV&AIDS status, they may also be compelled to disclose theirs. Their other concern is that they may suffer embarrassment if they disclose their family's status, and they are likely to lose a potential housemaid. Interestingly, employers' claim they do not ask about HIV&AIDS because they feel one would be intruding into the employees' privacy. Therefore, the less they know the riskier it is.

Many employers would want to see the attribute of *Botho* in their employees, and want the maids to demonstrate *botho* by disclosing their status however   if maids were HIV positive they are likely not to hire them. Ironically, they do not seem to want to extend the same conditions to maids. They argue that they would be putting their family at risk of being infected if they hire a maid who is infected.

Choice is generally at the centre of the decision-making process, and it ultimately influences one's behaviour and conduct. The different choices that one makes are mainly influenced by economic standing, especially in the provision of basic needs, and ultimately economic wants. The case of the maid is no exception. Food, clothing, and shelter are given priority, and where these are not available or are inadequate, individuals will go a long way to satisfy those first, including making risky, dangerous and suicidal choices. This is the position that housekeepers find themselves in, where the reality of providing for basic economic needs is to be made against the better judgment of dangers posed by HIV&AIDS.

Botho is a behavioural attitude that also influences the choices we make, and things a community is likely to be purchasing at household level, and ultimately at national level. Individual households' or firms' choices made at consumption level when aggregated become societal or national consumption, and in turn influence the national budget and income. Therefore, if *Botho* makes people to have mercy for those in need, it would make them expend towards alleviating the sufferings of others. In developing economies, such expenditure would generally be on such needs as housing, clothing, shelter, and food. These would not be attained if good employment is not created for people to earn an income. Employment opportunities of maids are as many as the number of households in the economy.

Maids generally come from low income or poverty stricken backgrounds, and that makes them venerable to exploitation. This means their education background is weak or poor. The link between poverty and HIV&AIDS prevalence has been debated worldwide, and there is some linkage.[1] Given the above circumstances both the house maid and the potential employer will make a decision that would apparently economically benefit them, which is not to disclose their status. It is this kind of decision that exposes the community to increased infections which in turn leads to increased national and individual expenses on the care and medication of the sick and ultimately the social responsibility to care for the orphaned in the event of parents' death. One is reminded of the following observation from the CRD weekly:

The Economic Impact of HIV

HIV is impacting on economic development throughout much of the developing world; as the UN report states 'By killing so many people in the prime of their lives, **AIDS** poses a serious threat to development. By reducing growth, weakening governance, destroying human capital, discouraging investment and eroding productivity, **AIDS** undermines countries' efforts to reduce **poverty** and im-

---

[1]Some studies and surveys have suggested that HIV&AIDS is most prevalent in the low income earning groups and the world continues the fight against poverty which directly affects developing nations.

prove living standards' (2). In some countries it has already caused a 5%increase in the number of people living in **poverty**, and in the hardest hit countries of sub-Saharan **Africa**, the gross domestic product may drop by 8% by 2010. Impoverished people are more likely to turn to prostitution, a tool for vival that increases their own, and others', risk of contract suring HIV. HIV-associated losses to the agricultural work force are resulting in lower food production in some areas. Around   7 million agricultural workers have died from **AIDS** in the 25 worst hit countries in **Africa**. Education services are also suffering staffing losses from an often low base. The disruption of families, communities, and social systems which result from famine, and violent conflict all magnify the impact of HIV, which is in itself destabilising. Migration for work, a norm in parts of southern **Africa**, also contributes to   spread through its disruption of family life. [2]

The definition of Human development, according to the Human

Development report 2004[3], is about the expansion and creation of choices in people's lives so they can lead the lives they value. Economic growth and power are therefore means of making the choices available. In exercising choice people must be free to participate in decision-making on matters that affect their lives, i.e. freedom of choice. It is therefore a human right to be afforded the opportunity to freely choose. An enabling environment where human development and human rights coexist is questionable in the above instance. The scenario in the survey does not seem to support the perceptions of securing the well being and dignity of all people, building self-respect, and the respect of others advocated for in the human development purviews.

---

[2]http://64.233.161.104/u/
hpa?q=cache:54mtcqdAW8cJ:www.hpa.org.uk/cdr/
PDFfiles2001cdr4801.pdf+Poverty+aids+infections+south+Africa&hl=
en&ie=UTF-8
[3]http://hdr.undp.org/hd/

Botho is about ensuring the humanity and respect of rights of other people. Why would people choose to deny themselves this noble notion? Economic empowerment is about extending and distributing wealth such that people can exercise choice. The challenge is whether the economic theory of choice, consumer behaviour, and utility theory are directly connected or influenced by behavioural change, *Botho* in this instance.

Why the Maid? HIV&AIDS and the Maid

The HIV&AIDS infection rate does not seem to be significantly declining, and this indicates that there are still behaviours within our community that have not been addressed. One such area is about the way we deal with our domestic workers. This stems partly from the stigmatization attached to the pandemic, and the mystic or taboo on discussions about the disease.

Every family, or at least a majority of families in major towns, cities, and villages have enjoyed or continue to enjoy the services of housemaids or housekeepers. Unlike their counterparts in government and corporations, housemaids do not seem to have the benefits that others enjoy. Yet, they remain a big part of our families. Those of us working for big corporations enjoy the benefits of being educated about HIV&AIDS and are afforded medical aid schemes that can buy us better health services and yet we do not extend similar benefits to housemaids.

New HIV&AIDS infections continue to occur despite the efforts made to change people's attitudes. Different education systems have embarked on various strategies with the aim to reach many, and thus warn them of the scourge.

- Could it be that we are addressing the wrong population if we do not address the maids directly?
- Could it be that caretakers in the formal set up (home-based care places) are more informed than others, and therefore better able to deal with their environment?

Notwithstanding all other duties of the maid, she prepares food for the family, cares for babies and the sick, but runs the risk of being infected, and of infecting other members of the family. When the maid takes up a job, does she get informed of the family's status, and does she ask of their HIV&AIDS status? What are the implications of such enquiries?

Without blaming the maids, they are in general very mobile, i.e. they move from one family to the other so often; they are generally low-income earners and the majority of them are least educated. They are thus vulnerable to abuse by their employers, and because they are socially and economically disadvantaged they are susceptible to manipulations by those who want their service and loyalty, unless supported by protective legislation. Even then, they may not exercise their rights because of fear and ignorance. How vulnerable are housemaid employers to the risky behaviours of the maid is clear for all to see even though many would like to turn a blind eye to the situation, and yet the maid remains a faithful integral part of our families.

In a survey, which we will discuss later, we found that maids are not generally asked about their HIV&AIDS status, and neither are they told about the status of the family where they are working. This has both economic and moral implications that need to be addressed. Secondly, there is no law that protects either them or the families where they work. The current strategy against HIV&AIDS does not address the maids as a sizable and strategically significant group of the population. This too has economic and moral implications.

Let me be the first to admit that I am no expert in these matters, but I was startled, and so were the participants (employers of housemaids) when they discovered that the questions asked in the survey we conducted were challenging their judgment, and showed that a threat they did not expect was by their doorstep. Many times, we distance ourselves from indirect problems, but are quick to react to problems when they affect us directly. When they present themselves at our doorsteps, we feel under pressure to address them. Often, we seek for quick methods to fix the situation; unfortunately, there is no quick fix for the HIV&AIDS problem.

Picture a situation where you leave your five-month old baby with a housemaid when you go to work, and think of the little games you play with the newly born. Naturally, as a mother you taste the food before you give it to the baby, you cut its finger nails, sometimes the baby sticks its hand in your mouth, then into its own. These are just a few of the things. Think of someone with HIV&AIDS who is not aware of the fact that they are infected, and loves and cares for your baby as much as you do, and does these little things.

You can also imagine a maid who has her own little baby she is suckling, who she leaves at her place every morning to come to work. It is no far-fetched speculation that the maid could easily breast feed your baby when she cries. You know the consequences if the maid has the virus. Note that she might be ignorant of her HIV status and she would breast feed your baby out of love.

The economic factors have been downplayed as secondary, but as we will argue, we observe that this was correct then, but we will show that nowadays it is not so. A typical middleclass mother has to work for a living. Given that in Botswana a larger proportion of the family household is headed by a female, and that children tend to be left under their mother's care for the better part of their childhood, who in turn solicit the help of a domestic worker, it is therefore important to look at the relationship between the family and the domestic worker.

The Survey
The results of the survey indicate that out of the sample population 93% of participants approached have engaged the services of maids. Only 1% of the participants had children that require maids' attention. All the participants did not enquire about the HIV&AIDS status of the maid for various reasons, the most popular being that it is a confidential matter, and they do not want to pry into the maid's private affairs, or be discriminative. It is such attitudes and positions that expose a vulnerable population to the dangers of infection.

On the other hand, maids do no not enquire about the HIV&AIDS status of the family they seek employment in. However, they would establish that no one in the family was seriously sick. This implies that maids use observations to determine if the family is infected. This analysis demonstrates how little informed the maids are. The data shows that 30% of the maids earned P200, and 37.5% earned P300. On average, a maid earned P300 for a 30-day month; therefore she got about US$1.00[4] per day. According to the 2004 UNDP living index, people earning this amount per day were classed as living in extreme poverty.

Conditions of the Maids Work

In all cases, the employers are covered by medical schemes, but all maids are not covered. The popular reason given for this is that the medical scheme has no provision for the maid, and maids cannot afford the contribution, if such a service were to be provided. Upon enquiry, insurance companies indicate that they have a policy that any individual can subscribe to for an additional person, and that is not specific for any person, therefore open to the maid. There are other benefits that some of the maids get, including free accommodation and two meals a day, but in some instances, such benefits are not available.

Apart from working conditions directly controlled by the maid's employer, there are financial, market, and economic conditions such as inflation and devaluation of currency that reduce the purchasing power of the workforce in general, including maids. Unfavorable consumer prices have a direct impact on the maids' income. The above therefore further reduces the real value of the maids' salary. Above all, the maids' power to negotiate or bargain for comfortable conditions is diminished by their lack of support from the revised National Policy on Employment, Incomes, Prices and Profits.

The workload of maids is somewhat of concern, since it does not seem to have definite boundaries and keeps being adjusted over time. Some of the maids expressed concerns that when employed they are briefed on what their duties are, but not all is revealed until

---

[4] Using the February 2004 commercial bank exchange rate

they have taken the job. They claim to be told they would do general house cleaning, washing, and cooking for members of the family. But they soon discover there is more in terms of the number and condition of family members than initially indicated, some of whom may be sick. When the employer is asked to come clean of the imbalances between the agreed and the actual situation, dismissal threats are raised. At this point, the maid finds it to be a waste of time to appeal for help, because the appeals process is long and the maids do not have the resources to spend on it. Therefore, they either give in, or resign so they can earn a living elsewhere.

The above are some of the conditions that demonstrate how vulnerable maids are to exploitation. In instances where an HIV&AIDS patient is home-based and cared for at home, the maid faces the real hardships of unforgiving risk of being infected while tending the sick. The risk is further compounded by her handling the patient without protection and providing other services such as washing and feeding other members of the family. Where an infected person is home-based, maids are not openly told, and when they do get told they are to keep house rules and not discuss family secrets, or risk expulsion.

The Maid

Many of the domestic workers are female and some are probably heading their own families. The domestic chores that a mother would generally perform is left to the maid, and therefore exposing children to many risky situations that may result from interacting with an infected person. Where a family member is infected, or the maid is infected, the reality is that infection is highly probable, unless this has been discussed and brought into the open by both parties to ensure that safety measures are taken. Practice shows that this does not happen for a variety of reasons, including economic pressure and the fear of knowing the truth.

The employer of the maid is under pressure to get the services of a maid so they can go to work, and not risk losing their jobs, given that job competition and the unemployment rate are high. On the other hand, the maid is prepared to take the job without question, fearing that an enquiry on the health status of the family may lead to losing the job. The age group of maids is generally between 18 and 30, and these are people at the prime of their lives. Quite a number of choices made at this stage determine a lot in terms of the life style they would lead. In this case, the economic benefits seem to determine the decision-making process.

The Middle Class Employer

We approached several middle class income earners to seek their views on the above issue. A Gaborone typical middle class individual in this case is measured by the style of life they lead, which is that they own or rent a medium cost house. They would own a car or two, use a gas or electric stove, have a fridge, own a television set and a VCR, have a land line telephone and a cell phone. They would generally not own all of these at one time, but have some of these possessions. While this may not be the absolute definition, we believe we came close enough to it.

Many of these people are degree holders, or hold a tertiary qualification and are employed in reputable organizations, with various benefits (car schemes, medical aid, insurance and education schemes) attached to their pay packages. We have tried to avoid using the actual income or take home amount to describe a middle class, but we used their life styles, as it seems to describe what they can afford.

HIV&AIDS as a Relations Problem

The maids find it difficult to discuss the HIV&AIDS problem because their interest is to get a job, keep it, and earn a living. Ironically, the process of earning a living may lead to a terminal infection in some instances. The AIDS problem has implications in the number of times that the infected person can get ill and the additional precautionary care necessary to guard against becoming ill. Those people employed in reputable companies, Government, parastatals and corporations seem to enjoy benefits through part contribution to medical schemes, although this may not be directly linked to the scourge. They also are given an opportunity to test and receive counseling and support from their organization.

The dilemma in this instance is that for example a working mother who has the responsibility and moral obligation to protect her newly born baby is forced to make an economically sound decision to either feed, cloth and maintain the baby having given up the job even temporarily or choose to engage a maid and not enquire about their HIV status thereby risking infection for her baby. Similarly, a maid who seeks to get a job, and not make any enquiry about the status of the family of the potential employer because they fear not getting the job is risking infection. Rationality is therefore brought to question—what is the rational thing to do?

Who should bear the responsibility? Is the maid's fear of not getting a job a result of the insensitivity or limited knowledge about HIV&AIDS by the potential employers? Or is the fear of knowing the HIV&AIDS status of the maid conveniently ignored by the employer to avoid accountability?   Should maids be put at risk because we do not want to pry into other people's confidential lives, or is it because we fear to disclose our status lest they become an open secret, known and discussed by neighbours and friends? Is it not our children and friends that would suffer because we failed to take a responsible decision in the contracting of maids?

As we begin to ask questions, we get close to home and a different picture emerges. People close doors because of the stigma attached to the disease, and the damage that it does to one's status and image within the community. While the disease cuts across class the different classes do not want to talk about it, and the infection continues. Class is once again determined by the economic well being of an individual. The irony in this is that the upper and middle classes will always seek the help of the lower class to do their poorly paid for and small odd jobs.

The suggestions herein are not an absolute solution, but they are seen as long term alternatives to address the infection rates. Maids and other domestic workers should be given free orientation of skills and ways to conduct job interviews. They have to be developed so that they can acquire the skills of getting information from potential employers during job interviews. Laws and modalities to enforce employment contracts with maids should be drawn, and a mandatory HIV test and disclosure to be made after the job offer has been made and accepted by both parties. We may not force people to stay in a relationship, but we can enact laws that compel or force the reneging party to compensate the other. In this case, whether some one is positive or not should not become a deciding factor, but should be declared so that precautions can be taken.

Humanity (*Botho*) versus Income Earning

The above conditions may sound too rigid and simple for a complex situation, but then why should the solution be complex? The situation here is one of give a little and get a lot, not in monetary terms. The cost of maintaining the sick through public hospitals and medication for HIV&AIDS related illnesses is drawn from public funds which is taxpayer's money. If we act responsibly we could save government's expenditure on this item. There are social benefits of a less costly and preventive exercise, with its foundations on the cultural roots of *Botho*. The nation will be a compassionate society that cares for the benefits of its lower class citizens and protecting them against the disease.

Can we say it is just a coincidence that the female population of Botswana has the higher percentage of those infected or it is just the proportionate representation since there are more females than males in the country? Has the infection pattern followed the nature of work that the majority of females are involved in, that is that of mothering and caring? Does the income pattern have a role in the infection pattern?

One cannot help wonder at the extent to which the spread of income and its distribution influence decision-making, where risk and choice are involved. The revised National Policy on Incomes, Employment, Prices and Profits passed in September 1990 (p24-25) left the issue of minimum wages to be negotiated between employee and employer, but where there is gross exploitation of wage earners, the authority should intervene. The negotiation between employee and employer has to be on a level playing ground. Unfortunately, the employer always has an upper hand, and is generally the controlling partner.

The report of the Presidential Commission on the review of incomes policy (March 1990) refers to the 1985/6 median monthly household incomes. The striking observations are that male-headed households were generally earning 20% more than female-headed ones, whereas urban male-headed families earn 32% more than female-headed ones, and rural male-headed households get 13.75% more than female-headed ones. Although there may be significant changes, the gender imbalance is still a reality. This observation is relevant, as house maids in this survey were heads of households.

The average household income at 1985/86 prices was reported to be P282 for urban households, and P132 for rural households. More than 10 years have passed since, and the economy has grown, but what the maids claim to be their monthly income does not reflect significantly on economic growth. The incomes policy has not compelled a minimum wage for the informal sector, and that has not helped much. The wages shown in this survey are far less than the 85/86 average, and have not grown with the economy.

Secondly, the distribution of incomes has not changed, where a smaller percentage of the population earnings are in the higher brackets, and a larger percentage of the population falls within the lower income brackets. The incomes gap in Botswana is a concern and closing the gap has remained a problem. Therefore the economically weak tend to be subjected to manipulation an attitude that does not help the HIV&AIDS problem especially for maids.

If HIV&AIDS infects a housemaid, two major problems are imminent. The breadwinners have their life terms reduced, and the dependants will suffer socially and economically. The alternative being that the dependants will depend heavily on the social structures and contribution of mercy. That is they will depend on the kindness of their relatives or the compassion of the society. Where the maid is not aware she has been infected and seeks employment in the next household, then the risk of infecting the next family is evidently high. It is therefore difficult for a society that practices *Botho* to equally discriminate against the infected.

Conclusion

This chapter raises concerns and shares sentiments of the public at large, raising issues of conflicting perceptions and ideologies. There is a dilemma as to moral practice and reality; the reality is that housemaids are expected to demonstrate the very best attributes of humanity and yet they are not afforded the same. They are to remain loyal even when they have to nurse an infected person in the family. If on the other hand the employer comes to know the maid is infected, then she is released or denied a job.

Without income, the infected maid is worse off. In the first instance, the survey found that the maids are forced by their economic positions to risk their lives in taking on jobs without checking the HIV&AIDS status of their employers and families. An employer also risks the life of his family by not making the same enquiry. This is the blind spot of humanity (*Botho*), which carries with it the human rights and respect. Humanity should not suggest ignoring the rights of the other person especially where one right interferes with the other.

Let us propose here that even if people have rights, whenever such rights impinge on other people's rights, then they cannot be upheld. For example in the case of the maid's right to privacy she also has the duty to protect the others just as the employer has the right not to disclose their HIV status to the maid but also has the duty to protect the maid against infection. *Botho* requires that both rights be respected by finding a balance between the two of them. A person who has the privilege of knowing other people's HIV status but later shares such information to the detriment of the other should be subjected to severe punishment. There is a need for dialogue about these issues with a view to coming up with a legislative instrument that can safeguard the rights of maids, and possible compensation for the risks they are exposed to.

References

Botswana Government (March 1990): Report of the commission on the review of the incomes policy. Gaborone.

Botswana Government (September 1990): The revised National Policy on Employment, Incomes, Prices and Profits. Gaborone

UNDP report (2004): Human Development report

Republic of Botswana: Labour Statistics 1996/7 Central Statistics Office, Gaborone

Republic of Botswana: National Accounting Statistics of Botswana 1974/75-1994/95 Central Statistics Office, Gaborone.

CHAPTER FOUR

The Significance of Cultural and Religious Understanding in the Fight against HIV&AIDS in Botswana

Abel B. Tabalaka

Introduction

Ever since the first cases of HIV&AIDS were reported in Botswana in the 1980's, there have been certain notions that people maintained in their interpretation of the HIV&AIDS problem. Most of these ideas were culturally and religiously-based. Examples of such notions include the following:

- AIDS is *boswagadi* (The result of having sexual intercourse with the spouse of a dead person before a purification ritual) (Botswana Traditional Religion)
- AIDS can be cured by traditional doctors (Botswana Traditional Religion) and through prayer (Christianity)
- HIV&AIDS is a punishment from God (Both BTR and Christianity)
- AIDS is a result of a spell or witchcraft (Botswana Traditional Religion)

Unfortunately, the believers of these cultural understandings were not given a platform to express themselves. They were instead lampooned and labelled as simply "mythical" and untrue. In their book, *Exploring Moral Issues in Botswana*, Kgathi G.L. *et al* (2000:31) classified the notions above under "Myths about HIV&AIDS." Kgathi and all who share her view continue to point out, "Because people are frightened of HIV&AIDS and do not know enough about it, they believe in stories about it which are not true (myths)." Thapelo et al (1999:16) also maintain this drift of considering the above notions as myths. It should be noted that the above sources are just a few examples from the pool of writers who have simply labelled these cultural notions as "mythical". It is of course very troubling to note that these sources did very little, if not nothing at all, to adequately study these understandings, their sources, and actually how these could help us in the fight against HIV&AIDS. The concept of *Botho*, which includes elements of rationality and morality, demands that we acknowledge the rationality in any given culture, despite how we may differ with its observations. Unfortunately, this was not the case with Batswana's cultural and religious understandings regarding HIV&AIDS. This chapter seeks to explore this problem and relate it to the *Batswana's* concept of *Botho*.

Religio-Cultural Understandings, a Stumbling Block in the Fight Against HIV&AIDS

Much has been written to demonstrate how cultural and religious misconceptions are actually a block in the fight against HIV&AIDS. Commenting on the contribution of African religion and culture on the spread of HIV&AIDS, Jon Lacey (2001) pointed out that culture and tradition can support certain extended relationship patterns and practices that may present risks of HIV&AIDS transmission. Lacey gives examples such as:

- early intercourse for males to demonstrate "manhood" (during and after initiation rites),
- genital mutilation (sometimes called female circumcision), and
- purification rites involving intercourse after the death of a husband.

In Botswana, this will be close to what is called *seantlo* (A Setswana practice where a widow marries her dead husband's brother or a widower marries his dead wife's sister). These, he argues may have some contribution on the spread of HIV&AIDS.

On the same note, Lesedi Mothibamele, who was the chairman of a Parliament's Select Committee on AIDS, said there was a need for cultural change, given the fact that AIDS threatens to wipe out the population of Botswana. This, he pointed out during the World AIDS day commemoration in Moshupa in 2000. Mothibamele argued that, "We are in a war situation where we have to make many tough decisions and forget about some of our cultural beliefs in order to save millions of lives," He said traditions such as *"seantlo"* must be discarded because they contributed to the spread of the disease (Daily News Online 5th December 2000).

The problem that arises here is on the possibility of "forgetting" or "discarding" these cultural notions, as the minister suggests. Is it possible to discard these without affecting other important foundational concepts of the people such as *Botho*? In other words, is it *Botho* to ask people to forget or discard their culture?

Myths versus Misconceptions

It is probably pertinent that before dealing with these notions, one should observe that a lot of injustice has been done not only against the ideas of the people, but even to the field of mythology. In other words, if for argument's sake we tentatively agree that the above statements made by Batswana were misconceptions; would we be doing justice to the field of mythology and anthropology by *labeling* misconceptions as myths? Are myths tantamount to misconceptions or nonsense statements? Probably this should be the first problem to be addressed. As Brunel (1992:ix) succinctly pointed out,

> The word myth as used today is loaded with much resonance and less meaning. Like other imprecise terms, it is used as an all-purpose word, particularly in the media […] it

has become laden with pejorative, petty significance and has come to mean advertent or inadvertent collective deception.

The problem discussed by Brunel is evident in the approach used by some in placing misconceptions on the same level as myths. It will be observed that this is of course a seriously problematic approach when we really want to understand myths. Although the word myths has been abused to a great extent, and overstretched even to the level of meaninglessness, myths are essentially reasonable. Putting it in Magesa's words,

> Myth constitutes a deliberate and conscious statement about society and man's place in it and the surrounding universe.
> (Magesa 1997:36-37).

Magesa argues that the language of myths is not an irrational form of expression. The only reason why myths seem irrational to some is because they generally use symbolic language, leaving a task to a concerned theologian to unearth and discover the understanding of such notions. In his definition of myths, Mbiti (1975:77) wrote that:

> A myth is a means of explaining some actual or imaginary reality, which is not adequately understood; and cannot be explained through normal description. Myths do not have to be taken literally, since they are not synonymous to facts. They are intended to communicate and form the basis for a working explanation about something.

From the above explanations, it will be clear that we cannot equate myths with misconceptions. These are two separate entities, whose essence and meaning cannot be linked. However, as we have already pointed out, the debate above should not be understood to mean that this chapter adheres to the view that the notions maintained by Batswana are nonsensical. Actually, the sentiments of this chapter are the opposite.

At this point, I want to demonstrate that contrary to the assertion of some, these understandings were developed neither out of absolute ignorance, nor out of panic and fear. One would undoubtedly agree that, using the apparatus of science, and having stayed around the HIV&AIDS problem for some years now, the accuracy of these notions has proved to be problematic. The fact is that it is not only the widows and widowers that are dying, but even children and elderly people (who did not necessarily lose a spouse through death) are dying from HIV&AIDS. Paradoxically however, this chapter seeks to depart a bit from the above drift, which is essentially simplistic in nature. Problematic as the understandings may be, it will be rather fallacious and actually frivolous to assume that people developed and hold this out of mere fear of HIV&AIDS, and out of ludicrousness. It will be clear that people already had some knowledge about related diseases, which they linked to HIV&AIDS. And this is the knowledge that this chapter maintains as necessary. To be able to show this, we will take only one notion and explore it. Although this chapter focuses on one notion, it is important to note that other notions follow logically from the understanding of the one discussed. For example, the fact that there is an understanding that HIV&AIDS is *boswagadi*, and that *boswagadi* could be healed through traditional medicine, that is, if noticed in time, it follows logically that people maintain another notion that AIDS could be healed by traditional doctors. Conclusively, these notions are then related.

AIDS is *Boswagadi*

The notion that AIDS is *boswagadi* is wide spread among many Batswana, especially the elderly people. Different researches, which were conducted among Batswana, have undoubtedly revealed this understanding. Besides Kgathi (2000) and Thapelo (1999), some important works include Molapisi (1995), Amanze (2002), and others.

According to Amanze (2002: 207-214), among the different tribes of Botswana, whenever a man or a woman lost a wife, he or she had to undergo certain rituals of purification. For example, one of the elders in the family went out to look for a traditional doctor who will be responsible to oversee the whole purification process. Moreover, the widow or the widower had to observe a number of stringent taboos for a particular period of time. Amanze points out that one of the restrictions of a widow or a widower is that he or she is not allowed to indulge in any sexual activity for a period of twelve months, that period is then followed by purification rituals. He argues that:

> Failure to observe this taboo can cause a disease called *boswagadi*. By most accounts *boswagadi* is considered the most dangerous disease among Batswana. Its symptoms are similar to those experienced by people suffering from the HIV&AIDS in modern Botswana.

From the above account, it will then be valid and very logical to point out that the notion by some Batswana that HIV&AIDS was *boswagadi* was not out of utter ignorance and stupidity. There is a form of logical association that a Motswana makes between the two phenomena. For example, Amanze outlines the symptoms of *boswagadi* as loss of body weight, coughing, darkening of the skin, failure to control one's bowels, just to mention a few. Most documented researches about HIV&AIDS would undoubtedly prove that the above listed symptoms are the same as the symptoms of a person suffering from HIV&AIDS. According to the Health Education Unit booklet, *Sexually Transmitted Disease* (1997:07), the symptoms of HIV&AIDS include, unexplained weight loss, diarrhoea lasting for more than four weeks, persistent dry cough, and unexplained fevers. It is clear from the above source that there is a close resemblance between the symptoms of *Boswagadi* and those of HIV&AIDS.

If Batswana reached the conclusion that AIDS is *boswagadi*, they are not making this statement out of utter silliness. They are informed by their prior experiences. They are making an association between the present phenomenon with the past phenomenon.

One important factor to note is that although some Batswana associate the HIV&AIDS phenomenon with the problem of *boswagadi*, they do not necessarily disdain its effects. As Molapisi succinctly observes:

> These people take AIDS as a serious disease as much as the problem of *boswagadi*. Although there are claims that they could heal *boswagadi*, they acknowledge that at a particular state, *boswagadi* is incurable, just as AIDS is incurable.

"Ke" as a Principle of Management

It is also pertinent for us to unpack the Setswana statement that "AIDS *ke boswagadi*" The Setswana word, *ke* can be used in different ways, such as in nominative, predicative, imperative, and copulative forms (Matumo1993: 139). Moreover, it should be noted that this word in Setswana is not used for subsuming one entity under another one, but a way of demonstrating a form of relationship. The word is used in the construction of phrases that demonstrate a relationship in character or nature of two entities. In Setswana, one can make a statement like, *"Monna yo ke tau"* (literally, this man "is" a lion). This implies that the man in question has behaviour or characteristics likened to those of a lion, but not necessarily that the man is a lion. This concept is called *Tswantshiso* (metaphor) in Setswana. It is a commonly used form of expression. I should hasten to argue that this type of expression, which we see used even when saying AIDS is *boswagadi* (AIDS *ke boswagadi*), is used for classifying, or categorising things in order to deal with them easily; it is a principle used for management; we name things and class them in order to adequately deal with them. The Batswana were thus logical in using this principle of management, especially when they were faced with a new phenomenon. It is necessary to categorize a phenomenon in order to develop strategies of better dealing with it.

The above principle is related to the important education system's strategy of taking learners from "the known" to the "unknown," or what is now known as cultural approaches to education. We cannot ignore what people already know, what they already hold, and try to take them into something new. This type of approach in overlooking what people know is tantamount to the irrelevant approach of some of the first missionaries who came to Africa with a mistaken notion that Africans had no knowledge of God. Hence, it was at times very difficult for them to penetrate into people's lives. We cannot expect any different results in the fight against HIV&AIDS if we choose to ignore the cultural and religious understandings of people.

Dealing with the Experiences of the People

Definitely then, if we want to come to the level of showing that AIDS is something different from the *boswagadi* problem, (which, scientifically is of course the case), we first need to acknowledge this factor. We are dealing with a mind that has taken time to make some logical comparison, and finally the conclusion. It is thus necessary to take time and efforts to show the difference that lies between the two. As already pointed out, a simplistic dismissal of such notions will be of no much help. The English saying, "Experience is the best teacher" should better inform those who deal with such notions, to realize that it is not necessarily going to be easy to simply obliterate such notions. As Peterson (1991:03) correctly points out,

> Religion is a very powerful force in human life [...]
> Evidence is abundant that human beings are incurably religious.

This factor is also made valid when observing that the notion above has an advantage of time; it emanates and exists within older avenues such as culture and customs of the people. Unlike the new information about AIDS, which is now being disseminated among people, these ideas have an advantage of prolonged existence in people's minds. People have been dealing with *boswagadi* in their culture probably from time immemorial. It is something that is part of their lives. Therefore, if some Batswana assume that HIV&AIDS is *boswagadi*, we should not take it for granted that we are dealing with a new thought. Although the phenomenon (HIV&AIDS) that is associated with *boswagadi* is comparatively new, the Motswana who is harbouring this notion is not seeing a new thing at all. He sees that old problem of *boswagadi*. Fighting an old experienced foe is undoubtedly very difficult.

Moreover, unlike the factual information about HIV&AIDS, which is foreign to the people, this notion is based on the tradition of the people; as such, it is more home-grown than foreign. I want to suggest that this is one of the factors that make these notions very difficult to erase from people's minds. As I pointed out earlier, the Setswana principle of *Botho* calls for an acknowledgement of rationality in every culture of the world. *Botho* thus demands that we acknowledge and appreciate people's experiences.

Conclusion

As a conclusion, one can point out that this chapter has demonstrated that people have their cultural understandings about HIV&AIDS. The chapter has attempted to demonstrate the logic behind these understandings. Although some attempts were made by some to try to obliterate these so called foolish ideas from the minds of the people without first understanding them, this chapter is a calling for an alternative strategy, that is a dialogue and co-participation between what is termed scientific knowledge and religio-cultural knowledge. By so doing, we will be adhering to our national principle of *Botho*, and we can thus expect some victory in terms of fighting the disease as a united front.

References

Amanze J.N. (2002). *African Traditional Religion and Culture in Botswana.* Pula Press; Gaborone, Botswana.

Brunel P.(ed.) (1992). *Comparison of Literary Myths, Heroes and Archetypes.* Routledge, London.

Daily news Online "First HIV case not taken seriously - Mothibamele," 05 December, 2000 <http://ccbux001.gov.bw/cgi-bin/ news.cgi?d=20001205>

Health Education Unit (1997). *Sexually Transmitted Diseases.* Government Printer, Gaborone, Botswana.

Kgathi G.L., Seganabeng R.R., Seretse T.E. (2000). *Exploring Moral Issues in Botswana.* Heinemann Botswana, Gaborone.

Lacey J. (2001). *Cultural, Religious Differences Contribute to African AIDS Crisi.* <http://www.newsroom.msu.edu/site/indexer/792/ content.htm>

Levi-Strauss, C. (1978). *Myth and Meaning.* Routledge, Britain.

Magesa L. (1997). *African Religion: The Moral Traditions of Abundant Life.* Orbis Books, Maryknoll, New York.

Matumo Z.I. (1993). Setswana English Setswana Dictionary. Macmillan Botswana, Gaborone.

Mbiti J. (1975). *Introduction to African Religion.* Heinemann, UK.

Molapisi K. (1995) *The Interaction Between the Theodicies of Traditional Religions and African Independent Churches: Focus on HIV/AIDS in Botswana.* (Unpublished)

Peterson M., Hasker W., Reichenbach B., Basinger D. (1991). *Reason and Religious Belief.* Oxford University Press, New York.

Thapelo B. et al., Morima N., Wills G. (1999). *Moral Education for Junior Secondary Schools.* Tasalls Publishing and Books, Mogoditshane.

CHAPTER FIVE

Methods used to Combat HIV&AIDS in Botswana: Implications for *Botho*

Sana K. Mmolai

Introduction

The introductory chapters have fully explored the concept of *Botho*. It is in the context of the foregoing that in this chapter we analyze the implications of the methods used to combat HIV&AIDS for *Botho*. Our aim in this chapter is to explore and establish how some of these methods may be understood to be contradicting *Botho*.

However, one might wish to define *Botho,* and most probably many would agree that the notion of *Botho* encompasses attempts to help others, or at least to desist from impeding the efforts of those who would like to help, and the attempts of those who need help to save themselves. This also applies in the case of HIV&AIDS prevention. *Botho* demands that all be involved in the combat against the disease. The question then is whether *Botho* would accept such combat even if it includes the sacrifice of *Botho* itself.

Put another way, does the combat against the disease mean everything is acceptable as long as it is in assistance of the fight? This is an open question, but one can ask whether there are methods of fighting the disease that are contrary to *Botho*, and if so, whether they are justified. Implications of the methods therefore need to be examined to determine this. It is also important to examine whether *Botho* impedes the fight against HIV&AIDS.

In this chapter, we will commence our discussion with the exploration of Abstinence as a method. As we shall argue, this method is based on one's ability to say 'NO' to sex. We will then proceed to examine Faithfulness as another method used to combat the HIV. We will conclude our discussion with the Condom, which, as we shall confirm, appears to be given priority over other methods by policy makers and stakeholders in our society today.

Abstinence

Abstinence is the decision to either delay or stop sexual activities. In some cultures, due to the orientation given in the context from which the principle of *Botho* has emerged, sexual intercourse is supposed to be delayed until marriage. In these societies, pre-marital sex was considered as a violation of *Botho*. To ensure that the principle was maintained, there was separation of boys and girls when they reached the stage of sexual activity. Girls remained at home doing household chores, while boys went out to the cattle post or were engaged in masculine jobs. For these young people, abstinence was not a conscious and deliberate decision, but was a part of the upbringing and orientation system that they had to comply with. There was no reference to abstinence among the adults, as marriages were arranged whenever children reached the stage of adulthood. It was uncommon for people to remain unmarried after having reached the stage of adulthood.

On the basis of this exposition, we realize that abstinence promotes *Botho*. To begin with, abstinence prevents unwanted teenage pregnancies, which no doubt contradicts *Botho*. It also promotes *Botho* because it is the ability to control one's sexual wants, by encouraging self-discipline. It further promotes *Botho* because, as already argued, young people who delay and avoid sexual activities before marriage are admired and viewed as well-mannered and self-disciplined individuals.

Abstinence from sexual relations before, outside, or in marriage does seem to have implications for *Botho* in the traditional culture. The most probable position would be that the Setswana traditional culture seems to have strongly disapproved of pre-marital sexual relations (Mmolai 1999). In which case, it would be against B*otho* for anyone to be either involved in, or encourage pre-marital sexual activity. It is however doubtful that abstinence was encouraged in marriage. This is because sex is one of the conjugal rights of marriage in this culture, which would be very difficult to deny someone especially a husband. This calls for a change in the sense of people rethinking conjugal rights.

The challenge here is to relate abstinence in marriage to conjugal rights in the presence of the dreadful disease. What does the teacher tell society so that it becomes informed and developed? The belief that by tradition married couples have to have sex would need a proper analysis and exposition. The following examples illustrate how abstinence can help in the fight against HIV&AIDS.

Young Matlhodi from Barotsi Primary School in Bobonong won the award for the best essay on her 'dream for the future,' based on Martin Luther King's famous saying, 'I have a dream […]' (Mokgosi, 2004:2). Matlhodi's dream is to become a nurse and educate Batswana about HIV&AIDS. Among the many issues she wishes to address would be to emphasize the need for young Batswana to abstain from sexual relationships before marriage. According to her, sex before marriage increases the risk of being infected, as it is not always easy to convince each other to go for testing. She would also encourage parents to educate and encourage their children to abstain from having sexual relationships before marriage. Matlhodi is of the view that the HIV&AIDS education in Botswana emphasizes the condom over both abstinence and faithfulness. One wonders why this is so! Central to the argument of this chapter is that, whilst abstinence and faithfulness promote *Botho*, condomization somehow impedes it.

Still on this issue, Pastor James Khanye of the Apostolic Faith Mission Church has been quoted arguing that gospel music has a great impact in the fight against HIV&AIDS, because it is against practices such as sex before marriage. It is believed that whoever takes the message of abstinence seriously can be saved from being infected, as confirmed by Pastor Khanye when he states that:

I also have some converts who I can say they are free from AIDS
because they are abstaining and waiting for their marriages.

(The Botswana Gazette, 2004:18).
During the launching of the HIV&AIDS Community Outreach
Project by Itekeng CJSS, head teacher Dirakano highlighted the
problems that his school faces that may contribute to HIV&AIDS
in the future. He said that there were some students who drop out
of school due to pregnancy, which according to him clearly shows
that students do not practice safe sex. Relevant to the argument of
this chapter is that Dirakano's concern clearly indicates that our
students do not abstain, hence their vulnerability in being infected
with the HIV virus.

If abstinence were given priority in our society, such incidents
of pregnant students would be unheard of. As we are all aware, it is
not *Botho* for students to drop out of school due to pregnancy or
any other cause related to sexual activity. This being the case,
abstinence would have been the best option. It is on the basis of this
fact that this section argues that abstinence promotes *Botho*. Frankly
speaking, whilst it is always *Botho* to be faithful and to abstain, the
use of a condom is characterised by negative factors, which impede
Botho.

Dirakano's concern about 'unsafe sex' confirms Keikotlhae's
(The Midweek Sun 2004:8) concern that in Botswana the **C**
component of the **ABC** (**A**bstain, **B**e Faithful and **C**ondomise)
campaign is given priority over the other methods. According to
Keikotlhae, abstinence is the only answer in our fight against
HIV&AIDS. His observation is that the **ABC** is a well-conceived
three-pronged approach that could prove worthy against the
pandemic in the long run. He, however, laments that it seems the
strategists missed the point by unnecessarily overemphasizing the
C component over the **A**. He observes that:

> The condom business has never been so lucrative. Condoms are
> tossed in the front at the expense of the best and effective measure
> of abstinence. The words abstinence and be faithful are mentioned
> but in passing amid the overwhelming publicity of 'condomise'. [...]
> We are not anywhere near the offensive against this pandemic but

only playing to the gallery. The real offensive is behavioural change, and change is an integral part of any society.
(Keikotlhae, 2004: 8).

As most of us are aware, in our Setswana culture, sex before marriage is taboo (Mmolai 1999). Perhaps it is high time we consider going back to our roots in order for us to be successful in fighting HIV&AIDS. Based on Keikotlhae's argument, it becomes evident that unless we change our behaviour and abstain, our fight against HIV&AIDS will be fruitless.

Faithfulness to one Partner

It would appear as if on the surface the *Setswana* traditional culture would advocate for faithfulness to one partner. This is in fact consistent with *Botho*. The problem is that it appears as if the traditional attitude has been that people can have extra-marital affairs, both sexes could have *dinyatsi* (concubines), only that it is considered *Botho* to respect one's spouse by not showing off their *nyatsi*, or disregarding their family and caring for the *nyatsi*.

However, one would venture to say that *nyatsi* was not something that people could actually be proud of. There was always a stigma attached to those practicing it, in which case the practice was actually contrary to *Botho* in the moral sense. Even though it was not outrightly immoral to have a *nyatsi*, it was not virtuous either. If this argument is correct then one can see the necessity to reinstate and infuse the virtue of marital faithfulness back into the traditional culture. It would also mean that *Botho* would demand that faithfulness not only be called for from wives only, but from husbands as well. The traditional attitude that '*monna ke selepe o a adimanwa*' (a man is an axe; people can exchange/share its use) or, *monna ga a botswe o tswa kae* (a man is not asked where he comes from when he gets home), should be discarded.

In this connection, according to the then specially elected member of Parliament, Shirley Segokgo, Batswana have to change their sexual behaviour if they were to successfully fight HIV &AIDS

(Sunday Tribune, 2004:2). Central to her argument is that multi-sexual partners are hazardous, irrespective of whether the act was practiced by men or women. Matlhodi concurs with Segokgo and argues that having multiple-sexual partners increases the spread of HIV&AIDS in this country (Mokgosi, 2004:2). Should she become a nurse, she would teach adults about the need to stick to one partner.

The concept of *Botho* is a vehicle through which the educator can convince the traditional Motswana that faithfulness is good not simply because it is dictated by the traditional culture, but also because it can save one from the dangers of HIV&AIDS. Whilst people could play around in the past, nowadays it is dangerous to do so. *Botho* does involve the need for people to take care of themselves and each other.

However, whilst there are people who are of the view that gospel music can somehow help in the fight against HIV&AIDS, lack of faithfulness by some religious leaders encourages other people to totally dismiss the effect of gospel music in the fight against the HIV/AIDS pandemic. For instance, Daniel Mogotsi is quoted as saying:

> I don't think gospel music can fight HIV&AIDS because pastors are highly involved in immoral acts like committing adultery and rape.
> (The Botswana Gazette, 2004 :18).

Mogotsi's observation indicates that it is *Botho* to be faithful, hence lack of respect for the religious leaders who commit adultery.

Because the traditional culture did not encourage pre-marital relations, it does not seem to make much sense to talk about faithfulness to one's partner outside marriage. This would then imply that the traditional culture would almost force people to get married. This raises the problem of individual freedom, and the right to decide how one leads their life. Bluntly put, whilst it is not proper *Botho* not to get married to someone one is willing to have sexual relations with, is it *Botho* for society to deny an individual the right to decide not to be married? In the context of the Setswana traditional culture, it could be *Botho* because the individual is basically important as a part of society, not as an independent entity. *Motho ke motho ka batho ba bangwe* (a person is a person through and with others) does not only mean that no person is an island, but it also means that the individual's importance is derived from the society in the sense of being intricately intertwined with it in such a way that the individual's importance is non-existent without it.

The challenge here is for the educator to reconcile or resolve the two conflicting moralities—the individual-based morality calling for individual rights and the community-based morality that calls for the respect of community rights at the detriment of individual rights. Which morality, if any, is consistent with the national vision of Botswana and why?

Condom

It has become evident in Botswana that it is unrealistic to suppose or even pretend that young people do not engage in sexual relations at an earlier age now than before. This happens despite parents' and some religions' attempts to prevent and oppose it. It also happens in spite of the traditional prohibition of premarital sex. Having realized the importance of sexual intercourse in the spread of the disease, and with the belief that abstinence is either difficult to achieve or simply not expedient for the modern day person, some people have called for the use of condoms as a method of controlling the spread of the disease.

Against this background, the implication is that the Setswana traditional view that parents should not talk about sexual matters with their young children has to be abandoned. Parents now have not only to talk about sex to their children, but they also have to teach them about the dangers of contracting the disease through sexual intercourse. They have to avail information about the protection derived from condoms, and probably teach them how to use condoms as well, because failure to do so would inevitably lead to children contracting the dreaded disease.

Two implications stand out here. The first is the idea that human beings are so desperate to have sex that they are helpless even under the threat of the disease. The question is the extent to which such a view can be sustained. If the urge to have sex is uncontrollable and that is against *Botho*, this would seem to imply that B*otho* should be done away with. If *Botho* has to be done away with, then there is the problem of convincing those who cannot envisage a Setswana society that is devoid of the traditional conception of *Botho* that it has to be changed.

The second implication is the necessity to abandon the traditional cultural norms relating to pre-marital sex, or at least to accept that they are so outdated that the only solution is to replace them with condomization. If condomization is regarded as not being *Botho*, then there is a problem in that the traditionally-oriented members of our society are not going to be easily won over to fight the disease on this particular front. This then becomes a challenge to educators. The challenge is twofold—to halt the ravages of this disease through education and appropriate behaviour change, and to convince everybody that condomization is the appropriate behaviour change from both traditional cultural morality and religious points of view.

The other factor relates to the distribution of condoms in Botswana. Since condoms are placed everywhere, for example in shops, refectories, everyone can have access to them, even school children. This results in children engaging in sexual intercourse at a very early stage, and that is not *Botho*, because they are not ready for sexual activities. Furthermore, the promotion of condom use may increase promiscuous sexual behaviour. For instance, people may tend to have multiple partners, knowing they would have 'safe sex'. In this context, the availability of condoms leads to unfaithfulness among married and unmarried partners, and this, as can be argued, contradicts *Botho*.

Furthermore, condoms are capable of empowering commercial sex workers, in the sense that they engage in their activities without fear of contacting the virus because they are protected. Arguably, the entire practice of commercial sex contradicts *Botho*, since there is no respect for one's body, as it is used for commercial purposes.

Another point concerns virginity. Culturally, Batswana placed great value on virginity. Young people were expected to remain virgins until marriage. To be a virgin was considered praiseworthy and honourable. This, as can be realized, is a sign of *Botho*, which condomization contradicts.

Amanze (2000) views the christian church's refusal to encourage its members to use condoms as a preventive measure against the contraction of HIV&AIDS like a "covenant with death", hence the title of his paper. He insists "the use of condoms should be a last resort when abstaining and being faithful to one's partner have failed." It is a lesser evil among several. He however acknowledges the fact that:

> the use of condoms in the fight against HIV/AIDS may consequently promote yet more promiscuity, prostitution and unfaithfulness that may eventually lead to breakdown of the morals of the social fabric, [...].
>
> (Amanze, 2000:207).

He believes that it is a realist position as opposed to the idealism portrayed by the Churches. This article is relevant to *Botho* in the sense that one may ask whether the principle of lesser evil is consistent with the concept. That is, if Amanze is right in arguing that insistence upon faithfulness and abstinence by the Churches is "a covenant with death," then the method of condomization as a strategy to fight HIV&AIDS is relevant and needs thorough examination.

There are billboards in the country that simply state that people should condomize to stay alive. Radio Botswana (RB 1) used to run such advertisements. Still related to this issue, the Botswana Amateur Boxing Association placed an advertisement in the Botswana Daily News (March 25, 2003 No. 57, p. 8). It was written boldly, **"TKO by proper condom use"**. The advertisement also stated that it was placed there for "the month of Youth against AIDS in partnership with the African Youth Alliance AYA." Here it is very clear that the campaign involves one of the methods for fighting the disease that we want to investigate—condom. The implication is there, but does the method cohere with the concept of *Botho*? If it does not, what is the implication for the campaign against HIV&AIDS? It could be that if people believe that condom use is inconsistent with *Botho*, then they are less likely to encourage its use. That might also affect their attitude towards the campaign against the disease itself. The message about the disease might be disregarded or not taken seriously. Such a state of affairs has moral consequences. The chapter wants this to be explored.

The national television station has also been running an advertisement that usually comes just before the nine o'clock evening news. The advertisement presents three gentlemen talking about HIV&AIDS infection. One describes a situation whereby a person can be infected. He says that a man can go to some place and meet a beautiful woman who could offer a beautiful sofa for bedding. This offer will result in the man being infected with the disease. The other gentleman says that cannot happen if one uses a condom. The gentleman repeatedly advises that one should use a condom.

There are two important issues related to *Botho* in the advertisement referred to. The first one is that the promotion of condomization is significant in the sense that it becomes pertinent to find out whether or not the condom as a method for fighting HIV&AIDS is consistent with the idea of *Botho*. Secondly, the advertisement gives the impression that it is beautiful women who transmit the disease—who infect unsuspecting greedy men. The fact that the advert is silent on whether or not men can transmit the disease and infect women is problematic morally. The question that arises then is whether or not it is consistent with *Botho* to campaign in such a way that prejudices are reinforced in the process of promoting a tool such as a condom. In short, is it *Botho* to campaign in such a way that gender sensitivities are non-existent?

It has to be emphasized while still at this point that *Botho* can somehow contribute to the spread of HIV/AIDS. To begin with, in

Setswana culture it is not *Botho* to ask your partner to use a condom. This request has two implications. The first implication is that you do not trust your partner, hence your reluctance to have "unsafe sex". The second implication is that you are not faithful; or rather, you are unsure of your HIV status. Either way, the use of a condom is suppressed by *Botho*. Furthermore, Setswana custom encourages men to marry younger women. In this context, *ga se botho* - it would not be *Botho* for the wife to ask the male counterpart to use a condom, since he would be older than her. This observation is further complicated by the fact that in the Setswana tradition, men have more say when it comes to matters relating to sexual relationships. As stated in the previous chapter, this cultural belief has negative consequences on the spread of HIV&AIDS in Botswana.

Another related issue is that young people are to respect elderly people. This being the case, it becomes difficult for a Motswana girl or young woman to ask an elderly partner to use a condom. Thus, whilst the use of a condom may be seen to be negatively affecting *Botho*, *Botho* can on the other hand contribute to the spread of HIV&AIDS by perpetuating inequality amongst men and women in matters pertaining to sexual relationships.

Botho can further contradict the use of a condom in the sense that culturally it is not *Botho* for a young person to educate adults on sexual matters. In this case, it would be difficult for a young person from Total Community Mobilisation (TCM) to present the issue of condomization to adults. Adults would naturally prefer someone of their age to address them. Another aspect is that many people consider morality before facing reality; for example, some people would be ashamed to go to clinics and ask for condoms, or even purchasing them from shops, in fear of being seen with such facilities.

However, having said that it could be argued that in a *Botho*-based society, people behave in such a way that there is hardly any need to consider condom use. But, in a society not *Botho*-based, it would not be "un-*Botho*" for the other party to ask for a condom.

The bottom line is that *Botho* should not have unreasonable or unjustifiable expectations on some people for the benefit of others. It can also be argued that condomization is actually not the easiest option of the three. Some people argue that for one to condomise, they need to abstain and be faithful. In this context, it is evident that suggesting condomization because the two are not applicable is not *Botho* because it portrays the irrationality of our action.

Conclusion

This chapter has analysed the implications of the methods used to combat HIV/AIDS for *Botho*. It has been demonstrated that generally, the implications of condomization, abstinence, and faithfulness to one's partner for *Botho* are too important to ignore. They need to be tackled by anyone who can have the least pretence to aspire for a developed and informed nation by the year 2016.

As has been argued, it would appear as if there is confusion or at least ambivalence towards the Setswana traditional culture. On the one hand, there is the acceptance that abstinence is good, which the traditional culture advocates, but on the other hand, there is the rejection of culture on this particular point on account of impracticality. The challenge is for the teacher to disentangle this complexity to the learner. This challenge actually provides an occasion or an opportunity for the teacher to gain experience in balancing what the cultural tradition demands as ideal virtue with pragmatic practicality. The educator has an opportunity to teach the nation resilience in the face of cultural irrelevance, de-culturalization, and epistemicide threatened by Western cultural imperialism. The challenge is balancing between the dangers of xenophobia and cultural intolerance on the one hand, and cultural annihilation on the other.

References

Amanze, J.N. (2000). *Covenant with death: the attitude of the Churches in Botswana towards the use of condoms by Christians, and its social implications. Botswana Notes and Records* "Covenant with death ... implications" Vol. 32, 2000; 201-208.

Botswana Daily News, March 25, 2003, No. 57, p.8.

Keikotlhae, C. (2004). "Abstinence is the answer in AIDS fight". In: *The Midweek Sun*, Wednesday July 28, 2004, p.8.

Odearly, A. (2002). *Beyong Condoms*. Plenum Publishers. New York.

Mathodi, O.D. (2004). "Ke tla fedisa AIDS". In: *Mokgosi, Mopitlo* 8-14, 2004, p.2.

Mmolai, S.K, (1999). *Religion and Ethics in Modern Education: A Case Study of Botswana.* (Unpuplished PhD thesis), University of Lancaster, Lancaster, UK.

The Midweek Sun, (2004). Itekeng CJSS CARES. DO YOU? In: *The Midweek Sun*, Wednesday March 10, 2004.

The Botswana Gazette (2004). "GOSPEL MUSIC: Can it fight AIDS"? In: *The Botswana Gazette*, Wednesday 7 April 2004, p.18.

Sunday Tribune, (2004). "Segokgo calls for behavioural change". In: *Sunday Tribune*, February 29, 2004, p.2.

The Concept of Botho and HIV&AIDS in Botswana

CHAPTER SIX

The Role of Religious Education in promoting *Botho*: Implications for the fight against HIV&AIDS

Joseph H. C. Mfuni

Introduction

The Botswana education system aims at developing *Botho*. An analysis of government documents on education reveals that one of the principle aims of education in Botswana is the development of people with acceptable moral behaviour. The important ideals, values, attitudes, knowledge, and skills that the education system imparts help to develop moral individuals. For instance, the report of the first National Commission on Education (Botswana Government, 1977) states that:

> In Botswana, education involves helping young men and women to absorb and understand the meaning of the national philosophy and principles and to build their characters and lives on the basis of these values. Becoming educated means acquiring confidence, skills, and abilities, and the capacity to persuade, organize and act; it means developing in aesthetic and moral sense.
>
> (p. 107).

This statement suggests that in Botswana the aim of education is not just to make people knowledgeable in specified disciplines or subjects, but also to make them develop *Botho*. As can be realized from the statement above, the aim of education in Botswana is to enable learners to acquire the qualities that can make them become moral human beings who, according to the Long Term Vision for Botswana (1997:12), possess high ethical standards. This means that the Botswana education system aims at producing educated people who are also morally and ethically upright.

Similarly, the report of the second National Commission on Education (Botswana Government, 1993) states that:

> The Botswana education system must help to develop people with moral and social values, cultural identity and self-esteem, good citizenship and desirable work ethics.

(p.5)

This statement implies that education has a crucial role to play in promoting *Botho*. From this it can be concluded that key to the aims of the education system in Botswana is to produce people with acceptable moral and social values. The same emphasis on the development of *Botho* is also reflected in the new Curriculum Blueprint for senior secondary schools. In this document, the government emphasizes the point that the education system should provide a foundation for a life-long education through the development of social and moral values (Botswana Government, 1998:6).

The role of Religious Education in the Fight against HIV&AIDS

Religion has tremendous motivational and inspirational potential to make significant contributions to people's values, attitudes, and behaviour (Watson, 1993:51). Because of this potential, religious education has always been part of the curricula for every education system. Even in the ancient Greek City state of Athens, religious education was included in the curriculum because of the contribution it made to moral development (Akinpelu, 1985). When Christian missionaries introduced Western education in Africa, religious education was part of the curriculum because it helped in the moral development of the learners (Makhulu, 1971:19).

In Botswana, religion has always been the basis of morality. Mmolai (1988) emphasizes this point when she states that:

> Batswana traditionally have a morality based on religion, even though the secularists and social trends are undermining it [...] In the 20th century Africa, ATR was undermined by Islam and Christianity. These religions also deal with ethical issues [...] (and) contribute to morality. (p. 23-24).

From this quotation, it can be concluded that since religious education can play a vital role in the fight against the spread of HIV&AIDS by promoting responsible sexual behaviour and inculcating the spirit of respect and compassion for those affected. In fact, it has been argued, from a moral point of view, that religious education is important because it provides the necessary conditions for morality. Yinger (1970), and Elias (1989) have argued that morality stems from religion. Similarly, Mmolai (1999:150) argues that in practice, religion supports and gives authoritative backing to the moral code. Thus, for one to be able to decide what conduct is right or wrong one needs a religious sensitivity. Such religious sensitivity, which comes form religious education (Meakin, 1879; Gardener, 1980), is of prime importance in the fight against HIV&AIDS and in the care of people with HIV&AIDS, as it makes people avoid sexual relations outside marriage on moral grounds rather than out of fear of contracting the disease.

Religious education has been made part of the curriculum so that learners may be taught not only to acquire knowledge about the HIV&AIDS pandemic, but that they may also learn about the responsible sexual behaviour that can help them avoid getting infected with HIV&AIDS. This chapter discusses the role that religious education plays in the development of *Botho*. It argues that since religious education promotes *Botho*, it can be used in the fight against the spread of HIV&AIDS by enforcing the message of responsible sexual behaviour, which can help control the spread of the disease.

Because religious education promotes such responsible sexual behaviours as abstinence and faithfulness, the objective is promoting *Botho*, as well as reinforcing the HIV&AIDS message. The discussion of the senior secondary school religious education syllabus that follows will further illustrate the fact that the religious education syllabus was designed to promote *Botho* among students.

The Aim of Senior Secondary School Religious Education Syllabus

The principal aim of the senior secondary school religious education syllabus is to enable students grow towards responsible Christian maturity, being able to see clearly the demands of their faith in their lives, and making their own values that they consider worthwhile (Chapman I, 1998:142).

The aim stresses the fact that this syllabus was designed with the intention of creating well-behaved persons who are capable of making responsible decisions and choices in the ever-changing society. In fact, the aim of the syllabus is in complete agreement with the current aims of the education system in Botswana. As stated earlier, both the 1977 and 1993 National Commissions on Education in Botswana stressed that the aim of education in Botswana should be to develop moral and social values in order to create people with desirable morals and ethics. This is exactly what the syllabus intends to achieve as it aims at promoting worthwhile values among learners.

Content of the Religious Education Syllabus

The religious education syllabus consists of five major themes, which are based on daily real-life situations. Using the life of our young students as a starting point, these themes include the Christian principles and values such as abstinence, faithfulness, love, care, compassion, etc - the values that are characteristic of *Botho*. These values are actually impressed upon the students as they explore the various themes of the syllabus. In this way, the syllabus can make a tremendous contribution to the fight against the spread of HIV&AIDS among school-going adolescent girls and boys. The following paragraphs attempt to describe how the characteristics of *Botho* are incorporated in the teaching of some of the themes in the syllabus.

The theme *Living in a Changing Society* has many areas where the characteristics of *Botho* are incorporated. For example, when discussing the *Ten Commandments* in Chapter 20 of the book of Exodus, the discussion of the commandment '*Thou shall not commit adultery*', involves explaining the implications of this commandment in everyday life. This commandment forbids sex outside marriage. It urges faithfulness for those who are married, and abstinence for those who are not married. The emphasis on abstinence and faithfulness can help encourage students to avoid sex and thereby prevent HIV infection. By abstaining from sex, students as young adults would be able to avoid contracting and spreading the virus.

The other related theme in which it is possible to incorporate characteristics of *Botho* is *Leisure in a Changing Society*. This theme provides the opportunity to discourage learners from getting involved in these leisure activities that may put them in danger of indulging in irresponsible sexual relationships, which might expose them to the risk of contracting HIV&AIDS. The students explore the ways of spending free time, and the problems associated with modern leisure activities. They discuss a number of leisure activities in which young people get involved these days. They learn about how leisure can be used to develop, build, and strengthen relationships. But, they also learn about the problems of new leisure activities. Facts about how they may contract HIV during these leisure times are stressed as they discuss leisure activities such as night mongering, beer drinking, and taking drugs.

The theme *Loyalty to Society* is about commitment. Students are taught that loyalty is about making commitments and remaining true to them (Chapman I, 1998:125). This theme also teaches young people about making wise decisions, such as abstaining from sex until marriage, and subsequently making the difficult choice of saying 'NO' to sex. In addition, the young are taught that in order to be able to make wise decisions and choices, they need to have independent thoughts or minds. This happens when they reach the highest level of loyalty. At this level, people make wise decisions based on intelligent personal initiatives (Chapman I, 1998: 128). This is what is needed for one to be able to espouse the preventive message of HIV&AIDS, and make the decision to abstain from sex outside marriage.

This theme also provides the opportunity to highlight the dangers of unfaithfulness in marriage. Topics like *Community Education* in the theme ***Family Life*** provide opportunities for incorporating basic facts about *Botho*. The whole traditional community was responsible for the education of the children. As noted earlier, children received training from infancy to puberty. Emphasis was placed on appropriate behaviour pertaining to a particular sex (Chapman II, 1998:54). When dealing with this topic, students can be allowed to discuss the sexual behaviours that show *Botho* and that help protect them from contracting HIV.

The African traditional family was the basic unit of society where people were loved, accepted, and cared for. There was the ideal of cooperation and co-responsibility. People worked together and helped each other. When considering these ideals of the traditional African family, the teacher may impress upon the students the correct attitudes that they should have towards people who are infected with HIV&AIDS. They can be taught to accept and love those who have HIV&AIDS.

The other topic in ***Family Life*** in which ideas of *Botho* are infused is polygamy. When learning about polygamy, students discuss the advantages and disadvantages of polygamy. Some of the disadvantages of polygamy are:

·   The problem of partiality on the part of the man,

·   The problem of older men going for younger women and hence depriving younger men of their rightful mates, and

·   The spread of sexually transmitted infections.

The teacher may emphasize these disadvantages and show how polygamy is against *Botho*. But, in view of the HIV&AIDS pandemic, the teacher must stress the danger of contracting HIV&AIDS as one of the disadvantages of polygamy.

Similarly, when discussing the topic S*ex Education* in the theme **Sex Differences and the Person**, the message about the responsible sexual behaviour that can help people not to get infected with HIV&AIDS can be infused. Like Community education in the theme **Family Life**, the topic *Sex Education* deals with the education that children receive in traditional society as they grow up into adults. Both girls and boys receive sex instruction and training during puberty initiation. This helps to instil proper values and responsible sexual behaviour for the adolescents (Chapman II, 1998:69). Consequently this helps to enforce the traditional codes of sexual behaviour that help to control illicit sex and teen-age pregnancies. When discussing this topic, emphasis on these ideals can go a long way in helping to control the spread of HIV&AIDS. Students may be given the opportunity to discuss the sexual behaviours that may lead them to contract HIV. Nowadays, young people have a lot of freedom and opportunity to meet and form friendships with people of the opposite sex. The danger is that this freedom of meeting and dating often leads them to engage in sexual relationships. This is why there is a need to make them aware of such dangers. When discussing these new courtship and dating patterns in the theme **Courtship and Marriage**, it is possible to teach them the characteristics of *Botho*, and advise them against engaging in sexual relationships. It is also possible to impress upon them the fact that they would be putting themselves at the risk of getting infected with HIV&AIDS if they engage in sexual relationships during dating and courtship. The teacher can advise the learners that they should abstain from sex until they are old enough to marry.

From the story of Gomer's unfaithfulness in Hosea 2, it is possible to argue that it is *Botho* to take back an unfaithful partner. But, in this era of HIV&AIDS, the teacher may use this story to expose the dangers of promiscuity as it might put one at risk of contracting HIV&AIDS. He or she may also stress the fact that reunion with an unfaithful spouse poses a moral dilemma. It might not be safe these days to reconcile with and remarry an unfaithful partner. This same argument can be made when discussing the stories about the woman who had many husbands, and the woman who was caught in adultery in the New Testament. In the book of John chapters 4 & 8 and Mark 10, Jesus condemns both adultery and divorce. But he advises married couples who have separated that:

> They should have courage to reconsider their relationships and to begin anew in the difficult process of loving faithfully and unselfishly.
>
> (Chapman II, 1998:82)

Such advice should be carefully examined in the light of the problem of HIV/AIDS. Students should be helped to realize that much as it is *Botho* to reconcile and remarry an unfaithful partner, it is not safe to be unfaithful in a relationship these days.

Methodology of Christian Living Today

The methodology of the senior secondary Religious Education syllabus involves discussing the various themes in the syllabus from a number of perspectives called *dimensions*. These include:
* The present situation,
* The African tradition, and
* Church history and the Bible

As noted earlier, this approach enables the students to consider a particular theme from a variety of experiences before they come to a conclusion in the synthesis. The students explore values from traditional African society, Church History, and the Bible and relate them to daily life situations in modern society. This leads to the synthesis whereby students have to choose an appropriate behaviour for their lives, guided by Christian principles and experience. The objective of this subsection is to demonstrate that the methodology of religious education can promote responsible sexual behaviour, which can help to control the spread of HIV&AIDS.

The present situation gives students the opportunity to take a closer look at the contemporary state of affairs regarding the matter under consideration. In this case, it enables them to recognize the seriousness of the HIV&AIDS epidemic in the world, and particularly in Botswana. They are able to see how the epidemic is capable of wiping out the population of the country if no steps are taken to control it. After looking at the current situation, the experiences of other people and their own experience, the students must be able to see the urgency of the situation, and come to the realization that there is need to heed the advice to practice *Botho* in our relationships in the face of the HIV&AIDS pandemic.

In the case of the theme ***Leisure in a changing society***, the lesson may start with an exploration of the many opportunities for leisure and the freedom of mobility that are there these days. The students may discuss how these can put them in danger of contracting HIV by considering the fact that leisure functions are usually held at night and away from homes, and that at these functions there is freedom for boys and girls to meet and mix freely. This exposes them to the danger of getting infected with HIV&AIDS, as there are chances of engaging in irresponsible sexual relationships. Moreover, some of the leisure activities that they engage in, like drinking beer and taking drugs may also place them at the risk of indulging in irresponsible sexual relationships.

The dimension of the African tradition takes the students back to Africa's past to see what the people did to control such sexually transmitted infections. Students learn that in traditional African society leisure was different from that of the society of today. Unlike what is the case today, in traditional society there was not much leisure, and there were very few occasions when people had leisure (Chapman I, 1998:58).

In addition, students may learn that in traditional African society leisure activities were held within the community and involved all people, both young and old. During these leisure times, traditional values and customs were taught and observed. For example, boys and girls were expected to behave in morally acceptable ways. They were not allowed to mix freely and indulge in love affairs (Mgadla, 1986:64). This left no room for boys and girls to engage in sexual relationships at leisure times.

Through the exploration of relevant traditional values and practices, such as the ones mentioned above, students get exposed to certain measures that were taken by people in the African tradition to control sexual activities among teenagers during leisure. They learn that these restrictions concerning the interaction between boys and girls, and the prohibition of sexual relationships between boys and girls, helped to control irresponsible sexual relationships among them. Building on the past ideals of the African traditional society, students may be equipped with the knowledge and the skills that can help them avoid engaging in sexual relationships and thereby avoid contracting HIV&AIDS.

Having explored the African tradition, students are then introduced to the way Christians in the history of the Church have responded to changing situations of similar urgency to the current HIV&AIDS epidemic. In this regard, students discuss how Christians helped to change situations at different times in the history of the Church. For example, in the theme *Leisure in a changing society*, students learn about how in the early centuries Christians helped to influence or change the attitudes of people from what were considered as bad leisure activities. This was achieved by use of good and interesting books, plays, and stories instead of the crude and cruel forms of leisure activities that prevailed at the time (Chapman I, 1998:69).

Some Church leaders, such as St Augustine, tried to keep Christians away from bad forms of entertainment by holding them up with Church activities. St Augustine used to keep Christians from undesirable entertainment by preaching extra-long sermons (Chapman I, 1998:69). When discussing this example, teachers may advise the students to keep themselves busy with religious activities so that they keep away from the leisure activities that may put them in danger of contracting HIV.

Students may also be introduced to the practice of renunciation whereby some Christians, such as monks and nuns, gave up certain things that they enjoyed. This may help students to realize that there are times in life when serious decisions have to be made to change their ways and life styles in order to avoid greater dangers. Emphasis should be on the fact that they should change their sexual behaviours so that they avoid the danger of contracting HIV.

Turning to the Bible, where emphasis is on the proper use of leisure time, students may learn about how the Israelites in the Old Testament times used leisure time to affirm their relationship with Yahweh, and to strengthen their relationship with each other (Chapman I, 1998:72). Like in the African traditional society, occasions of leisure in Jewish society were very few. They were limited to the Sabbath day, and such festive times as the festival of unleavened bread, the tabernacle, and the feast of weeks, which were characterized by sacrificial offerings and religious celebrations.

According to the commandment that instituted the Sabbath day, the purpose of leisure was to remember Yahweh, and to thank him for his goodness and to enjoy rest and fellowship (Chapman I, 1998:72; Deuteronomy 5:12-15). The commandment, which says *Remember the Sabbath day to keep it holy and in it you, your son, your daughter, your visitor, and your animals shall not work* (Exodus 20:8-11), suggests that the main purpose of leisure is to give people time to worship God and to relax with each other.

From the way Jesus spent his leisure time in the New Testament, it is clear that he understood leisure to be a time when one not only fulfils the needs of worship, but also enjoys rest, freedom and fellowship (Chapman I, 1998:75; Mark 2: 23-28). The teacher may use these ideals of leisure in the Bible to explain to students the fact that there is no room for irresponsible sexual behaviour during leisure. Students must be advised that it is abuse of leisure to indulge in behaviours such as sex, drugs, and alcohol during leisure time. To involve oneself in such things during leisure may actually put them at the risk of contracting HIV&AIDS.

The study of selected examples of stories from the Old and New Testaments may further expose the students to the experiences of people in the Bible who, faced with similar situations to theirs, tried to control their dire conditions by resolving to break away from unsafe habits and behaviours. The story about Hosea's unfaithful wife Gomer, in the theme *Courtship and Marriage*, is one such example. Gomer stopped prostitution and came back to her husband (Hosea 2). The other story is the one about a woman who was caught in adultery and agreed not to do it again (John 8). These stories teach the students that it is possible to change sexual behaviour. They teach that it is possible to change from a sexually active life to a life of abstinence from sex, until they are old enough to marry.

The fifth dimension of the Religious Education syllabus is the synthesis. This dimension gives a brief summary of the main ideas in each dimension and suggests the way forward. In this dimension, important conclusions are made on what has been discussed, and students discover the implications of these in their own lives. Students then choose appropriate behaviours for their lives, guided by the Christian principles. The teacher may use this opportunity to encourage students to choose to live a life of abstinence, and avoid irresponsible sexual relationships that may lead them to contract HIV.

Conclusion

This chapter has explored the ideas regarding the role of education in transmitting values, and promoting acceptable sexual behaviour in classical, traditional, and modern societies. It has shown that in the traditional African society, education was used for transmitting values associated with responsible sexual behaviour. This helped to reduce illicit sexual relationships amongst girls and boys.

It has also been argued that the Christian missionaries who introduced education in Africa ensured that religious education was part of the curriculum because of its contribution to moral development. It is against this background that religious education is still viewed as being a powerful tool for promoting moral behaviour, even in the current education system of Botswana.

The analysis of the aims, content, and methodology of the Religious Education syllabus has shown that the senior secondary school Religious Education syllabus has many areas in which the HIV&AIDS message can be infused. As has been demonstrated, it is possible to incorporate basic knowledge about HIV&AIDS in some of the topics of the Religious Education syllabus without necessarily having to review the syllabus.

Besides basic facts, it has been argued throughout this chapter that religious education lays emphasis on responsible sexual behaviour. This being the case, the subject is capable of helping the learners to abstain from sex before marriage. The major conclusion of this chapter is that religious education is capable of promoting *Botho*, and this can help control the spread of HIV&AIDS among girls and boys in Botswana secondary schools.

References
Akinpelu, J. (1985). *Introduction to Philosophy of Education*.Gaborone: Macmillan.

Botswana Government, (1977). *Report of the National Commission on Education*. Gaborone: Government Printer.

Botswana Government, (1993). *Report of the National Commission on Education*. Government Printer. Gaborone: Government Printer.

Botswana Government, (1997). *Long Term Vision for Botswana*. Gaborone: Government Printer.

Botswana Government, (1998). *Curriculum Blueprint for secondary schools*. Gaborone: Ministryof Education.

Chapman I, G. (1998). *Christian Living Today* (Book I). London:Cassells.

Chapman II, G. (1998). *Christian Living Today* (Book II). London: Cassells.

Dueteronomy 5: 12-15. *The Holy Bible: Southern African Tradition* (1980). Cape Town: Bible Society of South Africa.

Elias, J. (1989). *Moral Education: Secular and Religious*. Florida: Robert Krieger Publishing Company.

Exodus 20: 8-11. *The Holy Bible: Southern African Edition* (1980). Cape Town: Bible Society of South Africa.

Gardener, P. (1980). "How necessary is R.E".? *British Journal of Religious Education*, Vol. 3 (1), pp.66-70.

Hosea 2: 1-23. *The Holy Bible: Southern African Edition* (1980). Cape Town: Bible Society of South Africa.

John 4 & 8. *The Holy Bible: South African Edition* (1980). Cape Town: Bible Society of South Africa.

Makhulu, H. (1971). *Education Development and Nation Building in Independent Africa*. London: SCM Press.

Mark 2: 23-28; and Mark 10. *The Holy Bible: Southern African Edition* (1980). Cape Town: Bible   Society of South Africa.

Meakin, D. (1979). "The justification of Religious Education". In: *The British Journal of Religious Education*, Vol. 3 (1), pp. 49-55.

Mgadla, P. T. (1986). *Missionaries and Colonial Education among the Bangwato*: 1862-   1948). PhD Thesis, Boston University.

Mmolai, S. K. (1988). *Religious Education in Botswana Secondary Schools: Beginnings,Development and Future Prospects*. Unpublished MA Thesis, Lancaster: University of Lancaster.

Mmolai, S. K. (1999). *Religion and Ethics in Modern Secondary Schools: A caseStudy of Botswana.* Ph.D. Thesis. Lancaster, University of Lancaster: UK.

Watson, B. (1993). *The Effective Teaching of Religious Education.* London: Longman.

Yinger, J. (1970). *The Scientific Study of Religion.* London: Macmillan.

The Concept of Botho and HIV&AIDS in Botswana

CHAPTER SEVEN

Should Prospective Students Be Tested for HIV/AIDS Prior to Overseas Scholarship Grants? A Moral Perspective

Joseph B. R. Gaie

Introduction

There are many *Batswana* students studying abroad in countries such as Australia, Britain, Malaysia, India, China, Singapore, Belgium, Holland, Germany, France, Republic of Ireland, Canada, New Zealand, United States of America, and others. The students are pursuing both undergraduate and graduate degrees in various specialties. Many of the graduate and undergraduate degrees are not offered locally. For example, "Britain hosts 613 *Batswana* students" (Kebotsamang 2001:1) and there are 4090 students in South Africa (Motseta 2001:22)[1]. The quoted numbers refer only to government-sponsored students. Students in foreign countries are both government sponsored and non-government sponsored. For example, in April 2001 Debswana Diamond Company wanted applicants for scholarships tenable in "Australia, Botswana, South Africa, and the United Kingdom, depending on the course of study

---

[1]

	1999/2000	2000/2001
Local Institutions	13653	14944
Foreign Institutions	2729	5895

and availability of places (Debswana Diamond Company 2001:12)."[2] Botswana pays more for students studying outside the country than those in the country,

> The Ministry of Education will spend a whopping P167 894 500 in educating students in neighbouring South Africa in the current financial year.
>
> (Tutwane 2001:3).

This is more than twenty million British Pounds. South African institutions, however are less expensive than overseas ones.

> The minister explained that due to limited funds and the expensive nature of some Western universities, the ministry was avoiding placement of students in Britain, USA or Canada, except in exceptional cases.
>
> (Tutwane 2001:3).

An advertisement by the Student Placement and Welfare department reads,

> In view of budgetary constraints there will be no overseas placement of Ordinary Level Certificate candidates (O'level) in UK and USA.
>
> (Department of Student Placement and Welfare 2001:7).

> Britain hosts 613 *Batswana* students, who cost the government P95 million annually. The government spends an annual average of P155 000 on one student in Britain but only 15 000 for one at the University of Botswana.
>
> (Kebotsamang 2001:1)

---

[2]There are many parastatal and private company sponsored students. The University of Botswana, Botswana Telecommunications, Botswana Power Corporation, Debswana Diamond Company and Bamangwato Concession Limited are some of these companies.

It has been estimated that up to a third[3] of the people in Botswana were living with HIV/AIDS by 2001 even though this figure has been disputed.

> International organisations suggest that 38 percent of Botswana's 1.6 million people live with HIV, the virus that causes AIDS.
>
> (Matebele 2001:10).

From the above one may assume that those mostly affected by the pandemic are the most sexually active and those who are more involved in social activities. This group includes university students who get involved in risky behaviours (Siverts 2000:3).

The above figures actually raise the probability that HIV positive students could soon fall ill after completing their studies; or they might fall ill before completing their studies. If it happened that many students who were sent overseas for studies either did not complete their programmes or they died due to HIV/AIDS associated illnesses, what are the moral issues that may arise as a result? One of the questions that need to be answered is whether or not it is morally right to continue sending students overseas with taxpayers' money, in spite of the problems posed by the disease. One way of attempting an answer to this question is by testing the prospective students, and sending only those who are free from the disease. The question that then follows is whether or not such a strategy is moral, or should prospective students be tested for HIV/AIDS prior to granting scholarships? This is the question I seek to answer in this chapter. I am not asking whether sending students overseas in itself is morally right or wrong. That is a separate question, which is not the focus of this chapter.

---

[3] By 2007 this figure would have changed. 50 000 by 2005 would be on ARVS http://news.bbc.co.uk/2/hi/africa/4716553.stm. Last Updated: Tuesday, 26 July 2005, 03:50 GMT 04:50 UK

The issue of testing students and workers before studies and employment has been raised in Botswana by the media (Mogapi 2000:9), (Tsimane 2000b:30), (Motlaloso 2000:9). The University of Botswana Foundation and Botswana Insurance Fund Management (BIFM) organised a breakfast talk on the issue of testing students before scholarships approval, and workers before appointment.

(University of Botswana Newsletter 2000:1).

It is important, however, before proceeding with the discussion to point out that the availability of antiretroviral drugs (Mogale 2001:8) might shift the focus of the debate, so that it will no longer be taken for granted that when one is HIV positive one will progressively fall ill and die as a result of AIDS. The important issue would be, it seems, by how long the lives of the sufferers would be extended and what quality lives would they have, including the type of work they could do. Most probably, they would be able to do the work efficiently, and one would wish that there be hope that the next five years produce a cure for the disease, and the antiretroviral drugs could keep the sufferers until that time. The important point, however, is that antiretroviral drugs were not yet available to all people in this country[4] and most of Africa. In that case, if Botswana has to send students overseas, is it moral or

---

[4]By 2006 and 2007 many people had access to antiretroviral drugs in Botswana. Even then, the question of sending students who are HIV positive to overseas institutions still remains relevant from a moral point of view. Issues such as the availability of medical aid in foreign countries and the impact upon the national economy remain relevant.

immoral to demand that they be HIV negative? That is the question that needs to be answered. By "moral" I mean that it is right and should be done and by "immoral" I mean that it is wrong and should not be done.[5]

The question that arises from this title emanates from the word "should." The title may be understood to suggest that prospective students be tested for HIV/AIDS compulsorily, that is without their consent. It may also be understood to suggest that prospective students should be required to consent to undergo an HIV/AIDS test before they could be offered scholarships; meaning that the scholarship is made dependent on a negative HIV/AIDS test. It is in the latter sense that I wish to address the question. I start by saying that a compulsory test would probably violate people's human rights—the rights to privacy and confidentiality. It must be rejected for that reason.

It is expedient, at this juncture to define, though tentatively, what I mean by 'right'. I want to mean 'moral rights.' "Something that one can justifiably demand of others" (Gensler 1998:204). Rights can be described in terms of claims, powers, liberties, and immunities that people have (Almond 1993:262). Rights should be defined in terms of claims that demand respect. In our framework, rights are justified claims that individuals and groups can make upon others, or upon society. A right is thus analogous to property over which one has control, so that rights contrast with privileges, personal ideals, optional acts of charity, and the like. Legal rights are claims that are justified by legal principles and rules, and moral rights are claims that are justified by moral principles and rules. A moral right, then, is a justified claim, or entitlement, validated by moral principles or rules (Beauchamp and Childress 1989:56).

---

[5]I am quite aware of the fact that there are divergent views of morality. Some people think morality is subjective, others think it is the will of the strong and yet others think it is relative. The view I am advancing is against all these. The reasons are all debatable and would derail this debate.

The offer of scholarship on condition that the prospective candidate is HIV/AIDS negative can be morally justifiable on both Kantian (Kant 1991), and Utilitarian grounds (Gensler 1998:139ff; Mill 1991: 131ff). These philosophical positions are consistent with the *Setswana* traditional attitudes to life, as I will show below. It is also justifiable, on the basis of conventional practice, provided that practice is itself morally justifiable. This would mean that testing is morally justifiable in principle.

Compulsory Testing

The question as to whether or not prospective students should be compulsorily tested for HIV/AIDS before they are given scholarships touches on issues of human rights and professional morality. They are decisive in determining whether or not testing can be done with or without moral problems. I suggest that there are moral problems. By "compulsory testing." let us understand the case whereby one is tested against one's consent. Whether this is done by force or deception does not matter, but the crucial issue is the absence of consent. This has to be distinguished from the normal medical examinations routinely required from students before they are accepted into educational institutions, whereby they are not forced to undergo any medical procedures.

Supposing that persons or moral agents, have the moral right not to have their bodies invaded without their consent, then prospective students, as moral agents, have the right not to be forced to undergo a medical test, including that of HIV/AIDS. For anybody to forcibly[6] test the prospective students and claim that to be morally justifiable, they would have to show either that the prospective students do not have this right, or that there are other more morally weighted reasons which justify the impingement of the prospective students' right not to have their bodies invaded.

I contend that all people have the right not to have their bodies invaded without their consent, unless there is a weightier moral

---

[6]If one is tied with ropes and doctors are allowed to extract blood samples from them it is a kind of force.

reason. For example, rape is morally wrong because it is the violation of this right. It is a violation of the individual's right not to have their body invaded without their consent. Forcibly taking blood and urine samples and so on from an unwilling person is similar in kind to rape, only that the gravity of the violation may differ. So I think that the prospective students cannot have their bodies invaded through compulsory testing without violating their moral rights. For that reason, compulsory testing is morally wrong.

But, compulsory testing could be morally justifiable if there was a weightier moral reason.[7] That is to say, if confirming that the prospective students are HIV negative were a morally weightier reason than their right not to have their bodies invaded without their consent, then compulsory testing would be morally justifiable. My contention is that the prospective students' right to privacy and not to have their bodies invaded without their consent has more moral weight than the need to know their HIV/AIDS status. Therefore confirming the HIV status of prospective students against their will is morally wrong.

The foregoing has moral implications for the medical practitioner who would take the samples from unwilling people. In their professional capacities, medical practitioners have the duty to act in ways that are consistent with the aims of medicine. As a professional, the medical practitioner owes their allegiance to the patient. They are prohibited to use their medical knowledge for anything that is not consistent with the aims of medicine (Curran & Cascells 1980:224). In the case of a forcible test of prospective students, the doctor is clearly not in a patient-physician relation with the prospective student. So, the question is whether or not the doctor would be

---

[7]For example protection of society can be a morally weightier reason than the right of the individual not to be injected against their will or not to have samples taken from them without their consent, a mad person who has contacted Ebola for example, may be physically restrained if he or she refuses to be confined to a place where the disease would not spread and then injected with pacifying medicines to prevent the individual infecting the society.

doing what is consistent with the aims of medicine in testing an unwilling person, and my view is that they would not be behaving in a manner that is consistent with the aims of medicine. This is because the duty of a physician *qua* physician is to cater for the medical well being of their patients, both physical and psychological. A forceful test is not in tandem with the interest and well being of the patient (Amundsen 1978:23-30).

If one were to insist that the prospective student is a type of patient, albeit an unwilling one, then it can be shown that the doctor would be acting in violation of the aims of medicine if they tested somebody against his will. This is because the doctor's allegiance to their patient would demand that they side with the patient in case of a conflict between their patient and somebody else. So the doctor would ask the patient (prospective student) whether they want to be tested or not. If they do not want to be tested, the doctor would be morally bound to desist from testing the prospective student.

Offer of Sponsorship on Condition that the Prospective Candidates test HIV Negative

To begin with, it would seem to be important to point out that there is a moral distinction between testing for HIV/AIDS, and what is done following a positive result. It could be that in principle the testing itself is not morally wrong, the reaction or course of action following a positive result could be morally problematic, irrespective of the moral status of the idea of testing itself. Now, the question to ask here is whether or not the course of action following a positive result is morally acceptable. One view is that "one has a right (sic.) not to know their HIV status" and forcing someone to know their HIV status is "terribly wrong and unfair" (Letshabo 2001:12). I think the view is a misunderstanding. This is because prospective students can be tested without them necessarily knowing the results. All they could know, for example, is that their scholarship might not be successful due to the fact that they did not satisfy the condition that they be free from certain diseases including HIV and AIDS. Once that is communicated to the prospective students they do not have to know which of the diseases has been diagnosed. If they chose to find out, then they would not be forced to take that step.

I would like to urge that it is morally acceptable to test prospective students for HIV/AIDS, and offer scholarships on condition that the test be negative. This is different from suggesting what should happen to those who are found to be HIV positive. That is to say, if one is not offered a scholarship because one is HIV positive, that in itself does not dictate how onehould be treated.

Some people think that prospective students would have their rights violated if they were offered scholarships on condition that they test HIV negative (Matebele 2001:7). Joy Phumaphi holds this view (Mogapi 2000:9; University of Botswana Newletter 2000:1). Ditshwanelo, condemns the compulsory testing as a violation of human rights: "It violates their freedom from discrimination because it is impossible to test everyone in Botswana therefore the selection process must not be discriminatory." (sic.) Ditshwanelo said in a press statement (Matebele 2001:7). It is not a violation, but rather an impingement of the right, that is to say, a justified "violation" (Gaie 2000). What this means is that sometimes rights can be set aside or overridden because of certain justifiable reasons. Generally, people must be treated equally, but there are cases when discrimination is justifiable. One example is the preferential treatment for locals in consideration for certain posts, like the Staff Development Fellow at the University of Botswana. In such cases, the discrimination is justifiable and therefore not a violation but an impingement.

There are numerous cases of medical examinations before prospective students are registered in educational institutions, like the University of Botswana, Botswana College of Agriculture,

---

8 For example, on 27th February 1991 I went for a chest X ray as part of a medical examination required for acceptance into the University of Edinburgh. The medical certificate addressed "To Whom It May Concern," stated that I was medically examined and passed as fit to be employed for studies abroad. If I was not fit, most probably my studies would have been either delayed or forfeited.

Colleges of Education, and national health colleges. This practice seems to be international because of my experience with the universities of Essex, Edinburgh,[8] and Zimbabwe. Some employers, including the University of Botswana, usually insist on a medical examination before a prospective employee is allowed to take up a post. All these are forms of discrimination that may be justifiable.

Presumably, when these medical examinations are done some diseases such as tuberculosis would either delay the appointment or admission of a candidate, or cause its termination. Most probably, asthma sufferers would not be offered a job in the military, for example. Such discrimination is justifiable and therefore not a violation of any right. It is reported that,

> The Manual workers Union has taken exception to government and other employers who require people to undergo an HIV/AIDS test prior to taking up employment or going for further studies.
>
> (Motlaloso 2000:9).

The reasons given for such opposition are that those calling for people to be tested have not been tested themselves, and secondly,

> Unlike students, MPs who die of Aids (sic.) while they had been elected are given state funerals which are expensive. This means we should also test people who are going to be MPs or president.
>
> (Motlaloso 2000:9).

Whilst this is an important issue that needs discussion, it does not answer the question of whether or not testing students in itself is morally wrong. A quick response, however, to this argument is that it does not matter whether or not people have been tested. If it is right that students should be tested prior to overseas scholarships, it does not depend on whether those saying so have themselves been tested or not.

Joy Phumaphi is reported to have opposed the offer of a scholarship on condition that one is free from HIV because, firstly it violates people's rights, and secondly,

By resorting to compulsory testing, the nation would teach the youth that taking away people's rights was a solution for any problem.

(University of Botswana Newsletter 2000:1).

There are a couple of issues that need to be disentangled here. There is the question of testing every student before offer of sponsorship. There is the other issue of testing those who want to go overseas for studies. This paper is centred on the latter issue with the supposition that the moral arguments are different. Thirdly, the question of rights needs clarification—what particular rights are violated when students are required to undergo medical examinations before offer of sponsorships is not very clear from the statement. Bakuedi Masole is reported to have alleged,

Mandatory HIV testing is a violation of the fundamental human rights of the students—their right to confidentiality.

(Tsimane 2000b:30).

The issue that arises which many people do not seem to ask, and yet might be an assumption or an unstated premise, is that in the case of prospective students going overseas, they have the right to be educated. All qualifying students in Botswana equally have the right to be sent for further education. If that is true, it is not an unqualified sort of right. A lot of considerations, such as the availability of money and the ability of the student to finish the course and work, have to be made in order for the right to be granted.

More importantly, the prospective students do not simply have the right to education; they also have the duty to serve the country once they have that education. The state has the duty to ensure that, whilst providing the education, it is of the required type and the candidate is in a condition in which he or she will be able to fulfil certain obligations on completion of the studies. So, if HIV/AIDS was likely to prevent prospective students from completing their studies, or on completing them, if they were not likely to fulfil their obligations to work, the government would be justified in discriminating against those who are HIV/AIDS positive. The justification is that they are not likely to fulfil the conditions of their sponsorship, or put in other words, they are not going to be able to do what they were trained to do.[9]

The breach of confidentiality argument is weak to say the least. This is because when a prospective student is required to undergo an HIV test before offer of a sponsorship, he is not forced to have the test. The prospective student willingly undergoes the test in order to be sponsored. It would be a violation if he was tied or physically restrained and samples taken from him without his consent to such tests. Once the prospective student agrees to have the test, he also presents the results to the prospective sponsor. He is not forced to do this. He can choose not to divulge the information to a third party—a prospective sponsor. Once the prospective sponsor has the result, it is still within the limits of confidentiality, because he should not disclose the information to anybody without the consent of the prospective student. If indeed there was a breach of confidentiality, which I believe there is not, it has to be borne in mind that confidentiality is not absolute (Beauchamp & Childress 1989:335ff).

Utilitarian Justification

According to Utilitarianism, an act is morally right when it results in the most benefits for the highest number of people (Mill 1991:137). The maximization of pleasure or the minimization of pain to the greatest extent for the greatest number of people would be a morally good act. I am arguing here that this view can be used to support the argument that HIV/AIDS positive prospective students should not be sponsored for studies overseas. This is because the

---

[9] Here it has to be borne in mind that I am not advocating for the persecution of the HIV/AIDS positive people. There are many ways to engage them meaningfully besides sending them to overseas for studies they are not likely to complete. For example, instead of going for studies they could be given some projects that have more immediate results than a four to five year degree program.

consequences of sponsoring them result in worse situations for the students, their parents, relatives, and the government.

> AIDS reduces the benefits of investment in training for work and social growth (education). [...] those who died from AIDS (and who continue to die, usually soon after reaching their greatest creativity and productivity) were people with special skills, in whose education much time and money had been invested.
>
> (Bayley 1996:83).

This refers to a different country from Botswana. I am suggesting that if the statement is true about Botswana, then it is morally justifiable that the government stops investing in education if that is what the result is going to be. It seems to be true though that AIDS will impoverish the *Batswana* (Bungu 2000:17). The continued investment in education by the government would be immoral if people are not going to be better off than they are, as a result of the investment. This is how people are worse off. If government spends two million Pula on educating students overseas and at the end of three to five years the students either die or are incapacitated by AIDS, the people of Botswana would be worse off and therefore, according to Utilitarianism, it would be immoral if the government continued sending such students for training. This is because the money would have been taken from people's taxes, or from the country's investments, which arise out of such taxes. So, in monetary terms, Botswana would be worse off. The general population also becomes worse off because the fact that the money has been spent on the students means that the same amount has not been spent on the population. For example, lack of drugs and medical personnel could have been dealt with if the amount was available. Salary conditions of medical personnel could also have been improved.

If the majority of students are likely to die or be disabled because of HIV/AIDS before they are able to pay back society for their education, at least with services for which they were trained, then the students themselves would be worse off. This is because the money would have been lost, and the students would not be able to reap the benefits of their education. If the money spent on their training had been invested by the same student, and they were engaged in meaningful projects, the students would be better off even if they died in the end. This is because a short and happier, or less sorry life is morally better than a sorrier one of the same duration according to the doctrine of utility.

When students fall ill overseas because of HIV/AIDS, they are worse off than if they did whilst at home, where there is usually social support, which is important (Coser 1977:308). Studying overseas is not always an enjoyable venture. Above all, one is uprooted from family and friends while undergoing the demands of studying abroad (Mokgosi 2001:16). There is culture shock in some cases, and physical destabilization, including illnesses in others. These would impact more on an HIV/AIDS person than a healthy one. There could be better medical facilities overseas than in Botswana, but the overseas environment lacks the social support network that is available in Botswana. The attitude towards people living with HIV/AIDS, coupled with the belief and curiosity about Botswana being the hardest hit by the disease, can make one living with the disease uncomfortable. A student reports,

> Quite often I have been asked questions such as [...] how come your country seems well known for its high AIDS statistics? Are people interested in changing their attitudes in relation to their sexual habits or not? These questions are continuous and I must admit sometimes I do take a long time to answer.
>
> (Mokgosi 2001:16).

A sickly student in a university setting overseas is much lonelier than one who is at home, and is therefore more prone to pain and psychological torment than his or her counterpart who is at home.[10] Besides, a university student in Botswana can always call upon his or her relatives, or they can be called for him or her once he or she is not feeling well much easier than if he or she were overseas. It is expedient, however, to accept that the traditional social support system has at least changed a lot. Some people even talk of a breakdown (The Botswana Gazette 2000:10). But, it has not changed to the extent that can be comparable to the situation in the West. The Botswana Gazette (2000:10) speculates that HIV/AIDS is one of the reasons for the alarming rate of suicide, and is exacerbated by the breakdown of traditional support systems. If this is true, suicides might increase in the West, where the students are most likely to be left without the type of support that can be available at home.

It is also probable that students who fall ill while overseas will experience more psychological trauma than those at home. This is because the diagnosis of HIV/AIDS while one is overseas torments the student when he reflects on his life; especially that he has gone all the way, and for a long time in some cases, only to end up returning home on his deathbed. The thought that probably all the trouble of undergoing an education has come to nought would most probably trouble a patient, whereas other concerns would preoccupy a patient who is at home.

The anxiety, monetary loss, and anguish experienced by relatives and friends of a sick student who has to be brought home from overseas seem to be more intense, and therefore a morally worse prospect than when one is at home. It is painful for parents to learn that their son or daughter is ill somewhere in a foreign land,

---

[10]Baloi Thato who was the leader of the Botswana Student Union of the United Kingdom has argued that students studying overseas experience a lot of pressure and stress. He was commenting on the suicide of one Botswana student in another country. "Everyone studying away from home will concur that it can be extremely hard to cope. Many things are different and shocking, and as much as they can bring joy to others and they can bring mental disturbance to others to the extent that even the slightest problem be it social or academic can lead to wrong decision. This may seem light and easy to dismiss but many are depressed as a result (Thato, 2006)"

but they cannot come home because of lack of transport. For example,

> Critically ill Batswana students studying in the United States of America might die in that country if the Botswana government does not take urgent action to avoid having them ferried to the country as cargo. [...] American airlines are refusing to fly at least two Batswana students with full-blown AIDS back home.
>
> (Tsimane 2000a:2).

In 2006 Miss HIV Stigma Free 2005 got stranded in Canada because of illness, the fact became a media concern—the Midweek Sun wrote a commentary arguing that:

> To think that Leshomo is lying ill thousands of miles away from home, is a tortuous exercise. Obviously, this realisation affects the young woman negatively as she is constantly seized with the thought. Violence does not only manifest itself physically, but emotionally and psychologically as well. In fact, while the physical scars are able to heal with time, psychological wounds linger on forever. They serve as a memory to one's dark passage
>
> (The Sun Editor 2006).

Mmegi quoted her as having said "while I am sick from my own ailments, I am crushed by my stay here in a foreign land, with different tastes and cultures. I am getting worse not because of my disease but because of the environment" (Motlogelwa, 2006). Of course, these are perceptions that can influence the state of happiness of the people concerned.

So one would say that on Utilitarian grounds, pre-scholarship testing is morally acceptable in order to avoid experiences like those described above.

Kantian Justification

There is also a Kantian justification for demanding that students who go overseas for training be HIV negative. This is because, according to Immanuel Kant, whatever enhances human dignity is morally acceptable and a duty; whatever dehumanizes, or insults human dignity is morally objectionable. Immanuel Kant also holds that all people should be treated as ends in themselves and not as mere means (Kant 1991:95). I am arguing that sending HIV positive students overseas for studies when they are most likely to die dehumanises them. I also hold that the government and society at large have a duty to ensure that HIV positive students are not put in a situation in which their human dignity could be insulted. Society has a further duty to tell the students their moral responsibility, and the truth about their state. Failure to do that is tantamount to misleading them, thereby treating them merely as means rather than ends in themselves.

If the refusal by American airlines to transport the sick students to Botswana was actually true, we see that the human dignity of the patients was challenged (Tsimane 2000a:2). A human being has the right to be treated with respect. This does not seem to be the case when people are denied the right to be taken to where they would experience the love and concern of their families and friends. They probably are in this situation because the likelihood of it happening was not established before they were sent to these places.

Truth telling is important for a Kantian (Kant 1991:66ff).[11] It is therefore important to establish whether or not somebody is likely to complete his or her studies. If they go for studies with an HIV positive status the probability of completing their studies is low. Even if they manage to complete their studies, a further question would have to be answered truthfully, namely whether or not they would be able to fulfil the conditions of their sponsorship if they were HIV positive and managed to complete their studies. The condition of the sponsorship is that on completion of their studies they have to come back to Botswana and serve the country (Government of

---

[11]Kant holds that people ought to tell the truth even if the consequences of such truth telling are not desirable. What he means is that the justification for telling the truth is not that it is going to yield desirable results, but rather that it is the right thing to do in principle. If it is the right thing, in fact it should yield desirable results.

Botswana DSPW 4 2000:3-4), by carrying out the duties for which they were trained. The improbability of this being fulfilled when a prospective student is HIV positive is very high. It is therefore society's duty to make the student realize this truth and face life with it.

We have to realize as well that truth is liberative. It is only when people know their HIV status that they are able to behave responsibly, and in a morally acceptable manner. When the prospective student knows that he is HIV positive, he is able to face up to the truth that he could still live his life, and do something else without necessarily hoping that he could benefit from what almost certainly appears to be a dead end, if he goes for further studies without ascertaining his HIV status only to get ill and come back without having achieved much.[12]

The issue here is that there is a question of what is required of people when they enter into an agreement or contract.[13] Both parties have to be truthful. To be able to do that they need information that is material to their agreement. Taking the prospective student and their sponsor, the agreement is that the former must go for studies and come back to work for the country; that they are in a position, academically and health wise, to do so. The latter promises to cater for the needs of the prospective students whilst they are studying. The students have to fulfil their part. In the case of HIV/AIDS, the

---

[12]Of course, one may question the validity of this argument given the prospects of having antiretroviral drugs freely available to sufferers. At least up to the time of writing this chapter the government of Botswana did not have the means to avail these drugs to sufferers. It was the case with many African countries. By the time this book was getting ready to go to the press, the government of Botswana had managed to supply majority of its citizens with antiretroviral drugs. This did not include foreigners who had to pay for their medication. This development does not nullify the argument because even by 2007 the government still could not reach all its citizens with the drugs. It is also not clear if the host countries where the students went for their studies were ready to supply the drugs given their high prices in the West.

prospective students are not able to tell their prospective sponsors that they are in a position to carry out their part of the agreement if they do not know their HIV status. This means they cannot make that undertaking. To be able to say that they are in a position to undergo training and work for the country they have to provide their academic records and their medical reports. The latter can only be done if the prospective students are tested.

The reason why prospective students are usually required to undergo a medical examination is that they should be in a position to complete their studies without being disturbed by illnesses, at least the illnesses that can be detected earlier on. The Post Secondary bursaries or sponsorships Memorandum of Agreement explicitly states in 5.1(c) that the government may at any time terminate the agreement to sponsor a student,

> If Government receives a medical report which in its opinion indicates that the student shall be unable to complete the course because of illness.
>
> (Government of Botswana DSPW 4 2000:5-6).

Employers and educational institutions routinely require prospective employees and students to undergo and pass a tuberculosis test. The reason is that the two parties agree that the prospective student or employee does not suffer from a disease that may prevent them from carrying out their duties as students or employees. That undertaking cannot be genuinely made without the student or employee undergoing a medical test. Debswana Diamond Company placed an advertisement for scholarships in 2001. One of the conditions was that,

RECIPIENTS OF SCHOLARSHIP OFFERS WILL BE REQUIRED TO DEMONSTRATE A CURRENT CLEAR HEALTH STATUS WHICH

---

[13]All government-sponsored students in Botswana have to sign a "Post Secondary Bursaries/Sponsorship Memorandum of Agreement DSPW 4".

IS FREE FROM CHRONIC LIFE THREATENING CONDITIONS BY UNDERGOING A FULL MEDICAL EXAMINATION WHICH WILL INCLUDE AN HIV TEST.

(Debswana Diamond Company 2001:12).

This demand to employ people on the basis that they would not be prevented by disease from performing their duties is reasonable, and Kant would say that treating the prospective students as if they were not rational would be wrong, as that is below the dignity of a rational being. The prospective students have the right to say no to the test. If they do, as rational agents, they should be fully aware of the consequences of their decisions. If they do not want to be tested, it means the prospective sponsor would not be interested in sponsoring them. They should know this and be prepared to live with it.

One of the reasons against testing prospective students before being sent overseas for studies is the fact that they do not want to be tested for HIV/AIDS. The important question to ask in this regard is whether or not there is a Kantian argument for them to want the test. I submit that there is such an argument. Kant presents this argumnt in the following maxims:

> "To preserve one's life is a duty," and "to assure one's happiness is a duty (at least indirectly)."
>
> (Kant 1991:63-64).

From this, we can surmise that undergoing the test is necessary even if one were not intending to go overseas for studies. This is because if one wants to preserve one's life, one has to ensure that one is healthy. Ensuring one's health includes undergoing medical tests to determine one's health status, and to seek for medical attention if necessary. Arguably, it is better medically to determine the HIV status of an individual, since attempts at reducing the advance to full blown AIDS can be made, once the health status of the individual is known, than when it is not known.[14]

It would appear as well, to be the case that ensuring one's happiness cannot be by remaining ignorant of one's health status. This is because a rational being would not be happy to die in ignorance. Admittedly, a person may be distressed by the news that he is HIV positive, which is obviously not consistent with his happiness. But, it is difficult to say that a HIV positive person is happier if he does not know his health status. A rational person would rather want to know that he is HIV positive, so that he can prepare himself for whatever might result from that status. Having the right diet, desisting from certain behaviours such as smoking and drinking, doing enough exercise and getting counselling, would make one a happier patient than one who suffers in ignorance, and anxiety stemming from worries about whether one is HIV positive or not. Kant says,

> Every rational being must so act as if he [she] were through his maxims always a lawmaking member in the universal kingdom of ends. The formal principle of such maxims is 'So act as if your maxims always had to serve at the same time as a universal law (for all rational beings)'
>
> (Kant 1991:100).

To begin with, Kant believes that rational beings do not behave rationally when they lie. Lying to someone is disrespecting their rationality and therefore treating them merely as a means rather than an end. What all these mean is that the prospective sponsors should be willing to do what they would have done to themselves in a similar situation. This also applies to the prospective students. They should be willing to accept what they would do to prospective

---

[14]Nowadays there is the possibility of getting generic drugs to treat the disease even though there is no cure, which would be done if the person knew their status. So the fact that AIDS treatment drugs are expensive would not necessarily mean there is absolutely nothing that can be done by way of treatment.

students if they were the sponsors. When either of them fails to tell the truth, either by neglecting to find out the facts, or by wilfully deceiving the other party, they would be acting against the above Kantian principle.

Botho

The concept of *Botho* in the Botswana context is important. One may ask the question whether or not it is consistent with *botho* to advocate for offer of sponsorships on condition that the prospective student is HIV negative. My answer is in the affirmative. Before going any further, it is right to attempt a definition of the concept *Botho*, even though it is no easy task. This is because there is no English word that can capture the essence of this concept. Tentatively, we can understand *Botho* to mean morally ideal person, and conduct—fullness of virtue. A fuller definition has been done in Chapter Two of this book. The question we can ask then is whether pre-scholarship HIV testing reflects the fullness of virtue or not.

The *Batswana* usually say *nnete ga e senye botsala* (straight talk breaks no friendship). A person with *Botho* does not try to hide the truth, even if it is the kind of truth that is painful. When my mother, father, brother, sister, wife, or child dies, the *Batswana* insist that I have to be told. The same goes for a terminally ill patient. Traditionally, when a member of the family falls seriously ill, they are called and as they assemble, they are told the news. After that, a designated member is given the task of looking after the patient until such time that he is dead, or he recovers. This is important because it means people can be prepared in case a student is diagnosed HIV positive. The concept of an incurable disease is not foreign to the culture. In cases such as children suffering from fits, for example, the relatives have to be told so that they know *o a lwala* (he or she is ill), and therefore have to treat him or her as a patient.

Bogole ga bo tsalelwe (one does not have to be a cripple from birth—there are many things that can cripple a person), they say. This is important because *Botho* demands that people support each other when they are in trouble. Disability is not just a burden to the disabled person and their nuclear family. It is a societal problem. But first, people have to be in a position to know the disability of someone in order to help him. This is because there is nothing that can alienate a person from society, including disease.

Even though government and private companies might have signed contracts that enable them to discontinue their sponsorships of students when they fall ill because of AIDS, *Botho* demands that they should not abandon these people. That is well expressed by the fact that some companies have started providing their employees with free HIV/AIDS drugs. BP Botswana and Debswana have led the way (Dingake 2001:19; Malema 2001:23). I have to point out that this is possible now because the drugs have been offered for much lower prices than what has been the case before. This means that the service can be extended to students as well. This obviously means that the employees of these companies have to be tested for the disease in order to enjoy the benefit. It also means testing them prior to work cannot be a violation of their rights if it is intended to benefit them in the end.

Conclusion

It would appear that compulsory testing would be immoral as it is an invasion of one's privacy. It would also put medical personnel into a situation whereby they would violate the principles of medicine. This is different from the requirement that a negative HIV result be obtained before an offer of sponsorship is made. In this case, the candidate chooses to take the test because he wants to go for further studies. He is not compelled at all. This is justifiable on the grounds that it is common practice, and the practice seems to be reasonable. There are both Kantian and Utilitarian arguments for the test because according to Utilitarianism, it is more beneficial to have the students tested than not. Kant would say that human dignity is important for morality and that includes truth telling, which would necessitate the prospective students wanting to test as a matter of duty. Testing students is also consistent with the *Setswana* concept of *Botho*.

The Concept of Botho and HIV/AIDS in Botswana

References

Amundsen, D.W. (1978). *The Physician's obligation to prolong life.* Hastings Center Report 8 (4): 23-30.

Almond, B. (1993). *Rights.* In: A Companion to Ethics, edited by Peter Singer. Oxford: Blackwell.

Bayley, A. (1996). *One New Humanity the challenges of aids.* London: SPCK.

Beauchamp, T.L. and Childress, J. F. (1989). *Principles of Biomedical Ethics.* N.Y. & Oxford: Oxford University Press.

Bungu, J. (2000). *AIDS to increase poverty in Botswana.* The Midweek Sun. p.17.

Curran, W. J. and Cascells, W. (1980). The Ethics of Medical Participation in Capital Punishment by Intravenous Drug Injection. *New England Journal of Medicine* 302 (4) 226-230.

Debswana Diamond Company (2001). 2001 Scholarships. The Botswana Gazette.

Department of Student Placement and Welfare, Ministry of Education. (2001). Scholarship Application for 2001/2002. *Mmegi Monitor* 2(27) 6-7.

Dingake, K.O. (2001). HIV Policy In The Workplace-Debswana Leads The Way. *Mmegi Monitor* 2(23): 19.

Gaie, J.B.R. (2000). *The Ethics of Medical Involvement in Capital Punishment.* A Thesis submitted for the degree of Doctor of Philosophy. Colchester: University of Essex.

Gensler, H. J. (1998). *Ethics. A Contemporary Introduction.* London & N.Y.: Routledge.

Government of Botswana DSPW 4. (2000). Post Secondary Bursaries/ Sponsorship Memorandum of Agreement DSPW 4. Government of Botswana.

Kant, I. (1991). *The Moral Law. Groundwork of the Metaphysic of Morals.* (Translated by H.J. Paton). London & N.Y.: Routledge.

Kebotsamang, M. (2001). Return after study—Mogae. *Botswana Daily News,* (123):1.

Letshabo, M. L. (2000). Give HIV people a chance. *The Botswana Gazette.* P.12.

Lichtarowicz, A. (2005). Botswana Praised for AIDS Fight. British Broadcasting Corporation Health Reporter, Rio de Jenairo 2005. http://news.bbc.co.uk/2/hi/africa/4716553.stm.

Malema, P. (2001). BP Employees Get Free HIV/AIDS Treatment. *Mmegi Monitor,* 2(23):23.

Matebele, M. (2001). Mandatory HIV testing opposed. The Midweek Sun.

Mill, J. S. (1991). *On Liberty and Other Essays*, edited by John Gray. N.Y. & Oxford: Oxford University Press.

Mogale, T. (2001). Another US drug company slashes HIV drug prices. *The Botswana Gazette,* P.8.

MogapI, S. (2000). To Test for AIDS or not to test. *The Botswana Gazette,* P.9.

Motlaloso, S. (2000). Union Opposes HIV Testing For Jobs. *Mmegi Monitor,* P.9.

Motlogelwa, T. (2006). Leshomo sends SOS to Mogae. *Mmegi*, 23 (175) electronic version.

Motseta, S. (2001). Staff shortages blamed for Bursaries' woes. *Mmegi/ The Reporter*, 18 (10) p.22-23.

Siverts, S. (2000). Help Fight HIV/AIDS Individually and Collectively. *University of Botswana Newsletter,* P.3.

Sun Editor (2006). Editorial Comment. The Midweek Sun 12th March.

Thato, B. (2006). Morn the loss of life. In: *Mmegi* 23 (184) electronic version.

The Botswana Gazette. (2000). Alarming suicide rate points to breakdown in traditional support systems. *The Botswana Gazette.* P.10.

Tsimane, E. (2000a). Sick students stranded in US? *Mmegi/The Reporter,* 17(39)2.

Tsimane, E. (2000b). Testing students for HIV is discriminatory-BULGSA. *Mmegi/The Reporter,* P.30.

Tutwane, L. (2001). SA reaps education Ministry. *Mmegi/The Reporter* P.3.

Conclusion

Joseph B. R. Gaie

This book is not just about *Botho* as a concept. It is much more. It is an attempt at self definition of Batswana. It raises the question: who or what is Batswana? What identifies the pople of Botswana? Mmualefhe provides an answer, or at least part of an answer. Batswana are not only a part of the *Bantu*-speaking family of Africans, they are a people with a very rich language that yields a pertinent concept such as *Botho*, which is analyzable philosophically and theologically. It is a concept that is the very definition of what people are taken to be by Batswana. It is the kind of concept that needs to be unpacked. Even though the chapter does not say this; it is clear that our people have to be taught what it means to be a person from a Setswana perspective. It is only when we know who we are that we are able to ask others to acknowledge, recognize, and call us by name. Mmualefhe needs to be heard and understood to be asking these questions. It is an invitation to think in a Setswana way, which unfortunately has not been our strong point. People have actually adopted the habit of calling something Setswana-like when they mean it is inferior. The first chapter demonstrates that this cannot be sustained, and calls us to reflect on the stupendous possibilities open before us by our ancestors in our great language as defined by the concept of *Botho*.

The onslaught on inferiority complexes continues in the next chapter where I discussed the philosophy of *Botho*. Not only is the concept metaphysical, it is also ethical. What is more, the reader is invited to see the immorality of any suggestion that Setswana and Batswana do not belong or have nothing to say when philosophy is discussed. The Setswana concept of *Botho* puts Batswana up there at the high table of academic discourse; and also brings them down to earth where the speculative and transcendental is enveloped, and envelope the workaday practical situations. The concept of *Botho* does not just include epistemology, but there is a silent and yet loud and clear invitation to interrogate the concept, or to be instructed by it in all other areas of philosophy. This invitation is made to other areas—psychology, sociology, politics, economics, and so on albeit made in a manner that needs the reader to think beyond the paradigm.

Contrary to some of the Western conceptions of business and economics as the brutal exploitation of anything that is exploitable, *Botshelo* reflects the real meaning of *motho ke motho ka batho ba bangwe* (a person is a person through and with other people—not equivalent to no man is an island but richer), when he shows the interrelatedness of human beings in the face of HIV/AIDS. People might think that the poor, lowly housemaid is not important in the fight against the disease, and yet a lot is entrusted to them so that the way we treat them is not going to help us as a nation if we do not have *Botho*. This can only happen when we look beyond economic benefits and focus on what we are—being *Batho* (human beings) exhibiting *Botho*. The lesson is clear here; *Botho* is not just a theological and philosophical concept, it pervades the social and economic spheres as well. The power relationships between the maid and her employer are better served when there is *Botho*. *Botho* not only dictates that people should be treated fairly, it demands economic justice, which can be enabled by relevant legislation and good practice behaviours based on *Botho*.

Tabalaka reminds the reader of the presumptuous and pompous attitudes of Western type perspectives, regarding Setswana traditional attitudes to HIV&AIDS that are prevalent among our own people. There is a lack of appreciation of the cultural significance of language, resulting in some people thinking that others are ignorant and have no contribution to make to the struggle against HIV&AIDS. This turns out to be not only a sign of ignorance on the part of those who believe themselves to be informed, but also an impediment in finding a holistic solution to the HIV&AIDS problem. The lesson is clear—understand people's culture, know what they mean when they say something, and together you can talk from a common ground. This is demanded by the concept of *Botho*. It is a recognition, an awareness, and acknowledgement of the rationality of the local person. So listen, and listen carefully, and the Batswana will educate you and you will be able to see beyond their apparent ignorance and tap into their immense wisdom that has been garnered since *goo-Lowe* (from eternity).

Mmolai gives an apt demonstration of how the concept of *Botho* can be applied in our struggle against HIV&AIDS. What we are doing in attempting to fight the disease might be fruitless unless we appreciate the implications of that to *Botho*. For example, it could be that the apparent rejection of condoms by many Batswana is rooted in the traditional psyche that feels repulsed by current values. We have to reflect on these implications and do the morally right thing.

Mfuni argues that not only is religious education a potent tool in promoting *Botho*, which is morally required, but it also has positive implications for *Botho*. Making use of the school syllabus, he shows that there is a link between good religious education values and *Botho*, as well as behaviours that enhance the defenses against HIV infection, such as abstinence and faithfulness to one's partner. The reader is required here to reflect on the true nature and aim of education, and to see the critical role that *Botho* plays in all these.

Finally, the last chapter does not only show how philosophical theories of right and wrong can enable one to think what many dare not think in a rational manner, but also that the concept of *Botho* is an equally potent tool that can be used in the same manner.

We can conclude that this book is an invitation, rather than information, for the reader to take a maiden journey into the complexities of Setswana concept of *Botho*. The editors and authors would be happier if the reader realized the depth of the Setswana thought system, and ended up with more questions needing to be answered about this system rather than accepting their positions. It also states that we are here, and we want to be heard—our perspective as *Batswana* and Africans is important as a serious contribution to knowledge. For *Batswana* the question is clear: **what are you, and where are you going as a people? Are you going to globalize and lose your *Botho*, or are you going to make *Botho* your peculiar contribution to the global village?** The answer to this question is inescapable. Whichever way we answer it, we have to be aware that the answer is a matter of life and death for us, not only as individuals, groups, and families, but also as a nation, the continent, and indeed, as the whole of humanity.

Contributing Authors

Mr. Innocent S. Botshelo is a lecturer at the University of Botswana and holds a post Graduate Diploma in Financial and Business Economics from University of Essex and a Masters degree in Economics and Finance from University of Sheffield. He is a practicing educationist currently coordinating Business degree programmes offered by distance learning. His research interests are in distance and continuing education, economics of education, policy development and higher education management.

Dr Joseph B. R. Gaie is a Senior lecturer in the Department of Theology and Religious Studies at the University of Botswana. He teaches Ethics, Epistemology and Metaphysics based courses. He has written mainly in the area of Applied Ethics in which he subjects different behaviours to ethical examination. He is the author of *The Involvement of Medical Doctors in Capital Punishment: A Philosophical Discussion* by Kluwer Academic Press, now Springer, 2004. He is doing some research in indigenous philosophies and he is about to publish a moral education primary school textbook.

Mr JHC Mfuni is a Lecturer in the Department of Educational Foundations at Molepolole College of Education, Botswana. He possesses a BEd degree from the University of Malawi and MEd degree from the University of Botswana. His area of specialization is Religious Education. Mr Mfuni has extensive academic and administrative experience. He was a lecturer in Religious Studies and Educational Foundations at the University of Livingstonia, Malawi. He has served as a senior teacher and deputy Headteacher in a number of secondary schools in Malawi and Botswana. He has also served as an Examination Officer at Malawi National Examinations Board.

Dr Sana K. Mmolai is a lecturer in the Department of Languages and Social Sciences Education, University of Botswana. Dr Mmolai obtained her first degree and her Post Graduate Diploma in Education from the University of Botswana. She obtained her masters degree and her PhD from Lancaster University, majoring in Religious Education. She has taught for more than 20 years at the University of Botswana. She has participated in numerous workshops, seminars, conferences and projects on HIV/AIDS in Botswana. Her areas of interest include: the role of Religious Education in the fight against HIV/AIDS in Botswana, Faith Based Organizations' HIV Prevention Strategies; and Religious Education and the promotion of Botswana's Vision 2016. She is involved in a number of community development activities.

Rev. Dumi Oafeta Mmualefe is a lecturer in the Department of Theology and Religious Studies at the University of Botswana. Rev. Mmualefe obtained his first degree from the University of Botswana and his masters degree at Eden Theological Seminary in Saint Louis Missouri. He has been teaching at the University of Botswana for two years now and his area of interest include Christian ethics, contextual and practical theology. His research interest revolves around *Botho/Ubuntu* as a Christian discourse. Rev. Mmualefe, an ordained minister of the Congregational Church, is Southern Africa's representative in the International Association of Black Religions and Spiritualities and is a member of several learned societies.

Mr Abel B. Tabalaka is a Religious Education teacher at St Joseph's College and also teaches Epistemology and Ethics in the Department of Theology and Religious Studies at University of Botswana. Mr Tabalaka holds a BA degree and PGDE from the University of Botswana. He also holds a Dip in Pastoral Theology from the same institution and he is on the verge of completing his MA. He has written and published extensively. His research activities are generally centred on the theological and philosophical fields. Besides teaching, Mr Tabalaka is also an itinerary speaker and consultant in religious and academic institutions and is an influential local church minister.